Hajime Kojima · Troy Seidle
Horst Spielmann
Editors

Alternatives to Animal Testing

Proceedings of Asian Congress 2016

Editors
Hajime Kojima
National Institute of Health Sciences
Kawasaki, Kanagawa, Japan

Troy Seidle
Humane Society International
Montreal, QC, Canada

Horst Spielmann
Institut für Pharmazie
Free University of Berlin
Berlin, Germany

https://doi.org/10.1007/978-981-13-2447-5

Contents

Zebrafish, *Danio Rerio* as a Replacement Alternative Model Useful in CKDu Experiments

Mangala Gunatilake(✉)

Faculty of Medicine, Department of Physiology, University of Colombo, Colombo, Sri Lanka
mangalagunatilake@hotmail.com

Abstract. Zebrafish (*Danio rerio*) and its embryo has become a popular replacement alternative among the scientists because of many scientific attributes. As it is a model commonly used in ecotoxicology, our plan is to use this model to identify causative factors leading to chronic renal disease of unknown origin prevailing among poor, farming communities in Sri Lanka. This paper describes briefly the training underwent at University of Antwerp, Belgium and how zebrafish model could be used to address an important public health issue in Sri Lanka.

Keywords: Zebrafish · *Danio rerio* · Replacement alternative models CKDu

Introduction

The Concept of Replacement Alternative

Interest of scientists has been deviating since 20th century, from the use of animals in their experimental work towards substituting with 'Alternatives', thus reducing the use of live animals in experiments. This 'Alternative' concept is principally the 'Replacement' alternative that was indicated in the book; 'The Principles of Humane Experimental Technique' written by Russell and Burch in 1959. Although many methods of replacement have been developed and used by researchers, most of these are not **absolute** replacement models. As absolute replacement models should not involve whole animals and animal tissues, in many instances models used by researchers are **relative**. Relative replacement models include lower vertebrates, invertebrates or animals having lower level of sentience and tissues, cells, sera and embryos etc. of animal origin. These relative replacement models of course reduce or prevent the use of conscious living vertebrates [1].

Scientific Importance of Zebrafish *(Danio Rerio)*

Among the accepted relative replacement models, the zebrafish (ZF) and its embryo model have been of interest to the researchers due to its wide spectrum of scientific applicability. ZF and its embryo have been used in diverse fields of science including

H. Kojima et al. (Eds.): *Alternatives to Animal Testing*, pp. 1–7, 2019.
https://doi.org/10.1007/978-981-13-2447-5_1

developmental biology, oncology, pharmacology, toxicology, teratology, genetics, neurobiology, environmental sciences, stem cell research etc. [2–6]. Identification of substances/key molecules responsible for regenerative capacity of damaged heart muscle, retinal tissues of eyes, nerve fibers shed light for the scientists one day to focus on new therapies for people with ischaemic heart disease, spinal cord injuries and to combat degenerative eye disease damage in humans [7–9].

Scientific Attributes of Zebrafish

ZF, specially its embryo model has its wide acceptance and popularity as a replacement model due to many scientific attributes such as small size of ZF, ease of maintenance, low cost, rapid growth rate, high fecundity rate, external fertilization, optical transparency of the embryo (Figs. 1 and 2), ease of genetic manipulations, high genetic similarity to humans and regenerative capacity [2, 5].

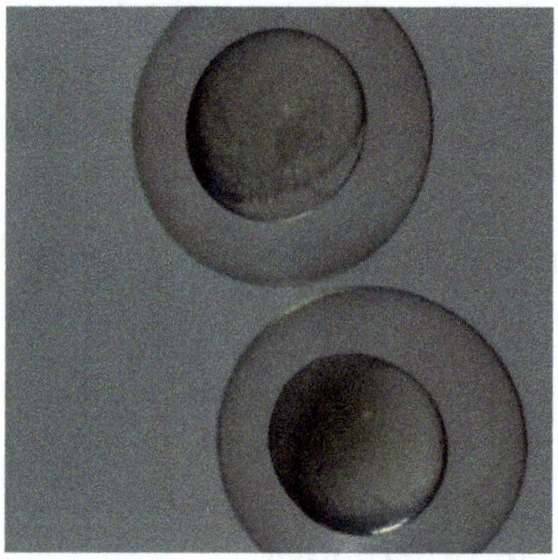

Fig. 1. Normal embryos after collection (Inverted microscope-Leica 10447137 model 10X/23, X1.0)

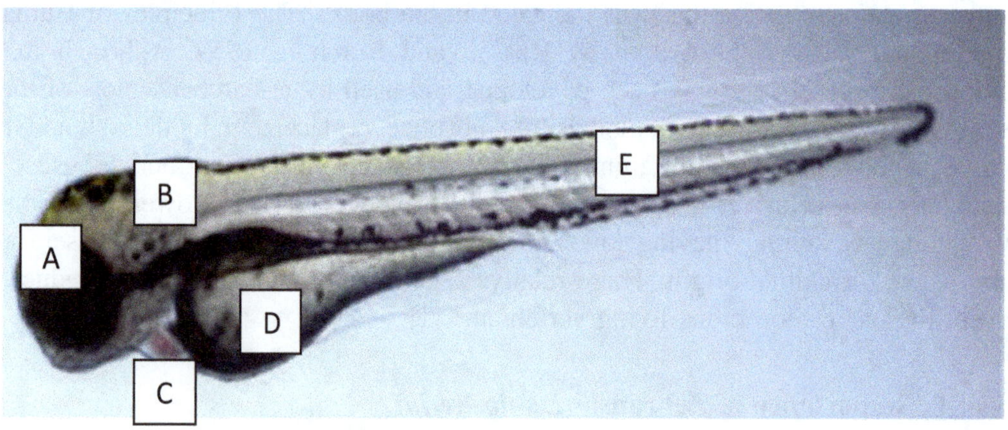

Fig. 2. Normal Zebrafish embryo at 72 hpf. (Inverted microscope-Leica 10447137 model 10X/23, X2.0). A: Eyes, B: Otoloths, C: Heart, D: Yolk sac and its extension, E: Vertebral coloumn

Introduction of Zebrafish Model to Sri Lanka

Scientific benefits of ZF and its embryo was unknown to most of Sri Lankan researchers until its introduction to Sri Lankans at the Inaugural Scientific Conference of the Sri Lanka Association for Laboratory Animal Science (SLALAS) in January 2014 by Dr. Francois Busquet, CAAT-Europe Policy Coordinator, University of Konstanz, Germany. ZF, which is a native species in Sri Lanka, is used as an ornamental fish [10]. The wild type and ZF in different colours, produced through genetic manipulations by the breeders, are available in Sri Lankan aquaria for this purpose.

Materials and Methods

Comprehensive Training on Zebrafish Model

Transparency of the developing ZF embryo during demonstrations at the Inaugural Conference of SLALAS was very impressive and an eye opener for most of Sri Lankan researchers to concentrate on replacement alternatives. This created an interest for acquisition of more knowledge and skills on ZF embryo model. Thus a 2-week comprehensive training at the ZF lab in University of Antwerp, Belgium was possible because of the Overseas Special Training Fellowship granted by the National Science Foundation of Sri Lanka. The material such as ZF embryos, testing chemicals, inverted microscopic facilities with recording of images etc. needed during training was kindly provided by Prof. Dries Knapen, Head of the ZF lab of University of Antwerp through the research grants secured by him.

During this 2-week training, the principal focus was on three areas.

1. Operation and daily maintenance of the ZF housing facility provided an insight in to different housing systems; fully automated standalone, semi-automated tanking and aquarium type housing systems that could be established in a ZF lab depending on the financial capacities. Hands-on was possible on the frequency and method of water quality testing for pH, temperature, salinity/conductivity and hardness of water, which are prerequisites for reproduction, and maintenance of fish in the tanks. It was also emphasized the need for different types of filters; chemical, biological and UV. Maintenance of good standards improves quality of research procedures and reproducibility of research data.
2. Daily maintenance and reproduction of ZF in practice covered nutritional requirements of ZF at different stages of growth, feeding patterns and need for variation in food types. In order to use ZF embryo as a research model, knowledge on how to facilitate spawning, collection of eggs, selection of good quality eggs are essential, and thus practiced.
3. Standardized morphological scoring of ZF embryos and larvae as an important item during training gave an insight in to how ZF embryo could be used for water quality testing and acute toxicity testing of substances according to ISO 15088:2007 and OECD guideline 236 [11–13]. Two concentrations; 600 mM and 1200 mM of caffeine (Kofeina, 1, 3, 7-Trimethylxanthine, Sigma Aldrich) were used during practice. When performing this test, newly fertilized ZF eggs (n = 60 per sample

solution) in water samples different concentrations of toxic substances for a period of 96 h (96 h post fertilization—96 hpf), with positive (3, 4-Dichlore aniline) and negative control solutions should be incubated. Observations with an inverted microscope at every 24 h are needed to identify the four endpoints; coagulation of fertilized eggs, lack of somite formation, lack of detachment of the tail-bud from the yolk sac (Figs. 3, 4 and 5), lack of heartbeat. At the end of the exposure period, determination of acute toxicity could be done based on a positive outcome in any of the above mentioned recorded observations leading to calculation of LC50 value.

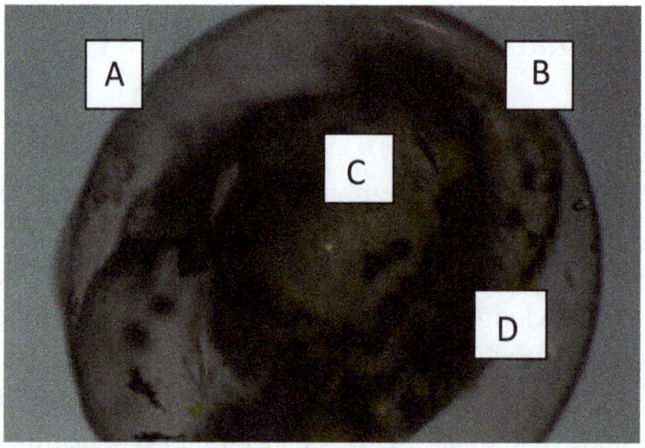

Fig. 3. At 72 hpf of exposure to 1200 mM of caffeine Solution. (Inverted microscope-Leica 10447137 model 10X/23, X3.0). A: Embryo is not hatched, B: Non detachment of the tail, C: Presence of severe edema in the developing embryo and D: Lack of somite formation

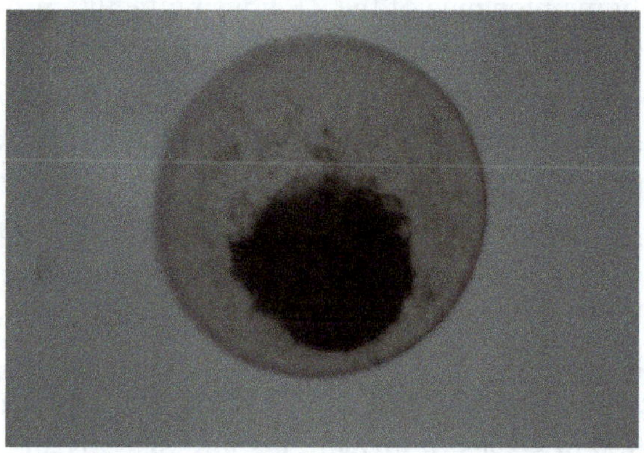

Fig. 4. Coagulated embryo (Inverted microscope-Leica 10447137 model 10X/23, X1.0)

Results

In addition to four end-points of acute toxicity test, abnormalities such as malformation of tail, pectoral fin, yolk sac, head, eyes, otoliths, mouth and heart; pericardial and yolk sac edema, accumulation of blood, disturbed or no blood flow in the tail; abnormal pigmentation; non-detachment of tail and un-inflated swim bladder leading to abnormal

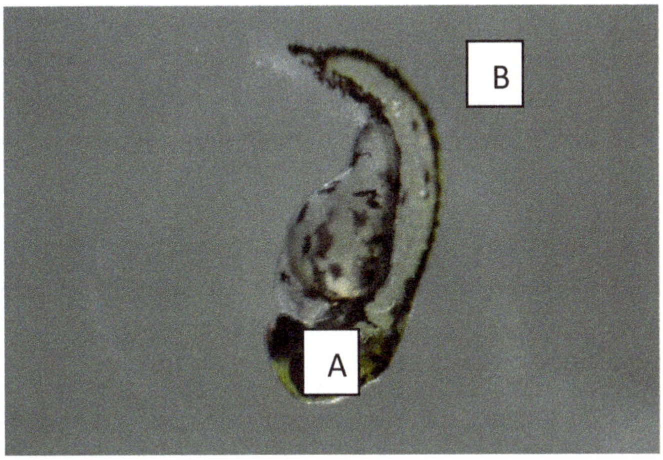

Fig. 5. At 72 hpf- Abnormal larvae. (Inverted microscope-Leica 10447137 model 10X/23, X1.0) A: Percardial edema, B: Curved tail.

movements of larvae, were also observed during this training. Necessity for adoption of a scoring system to quantify observations for scientific presentation of data was emphasized.

When using ZF model in experimental procedures the need for ethics and welfare aspects too need to be considered. It is accepted that ZF larvae develops the capability in independent feeding without depending on the food supply from the yolk sac and feeling of pain sensation around 120 hpf (Drs. An Hagenaars and Lucia Vergauwen of Zebrafish lab, University of Antwerp- Personnel communication during training, [14]). Therefore, the need for ethics approval for the use of ZF embryo in acute toxicity testing does not arise.

Discussion and Conclusion

Acute toxicity test with ZF embryo as a replacement alternative has become the easiest and most convenient test because the test could be performed within 4 days of post fertilization (96 hpf) without breaching ethics and welfare. However, there are several tests where ZF can be used subjected to ethics approval. ZF model has a wide spectrum of applicability in the Sri Lankan context instead of rodents and rabbits thus the application of 3Rs concept in the experimental procedures.

Scientific Applicability of Zebrafish Model in the Sri Lankan Context

Being a fresh water fish, ZF and its developing stages are sensitive to changes in their immediate environment [15]. These changes could cause mortality, and also affects all their activities and growth in developing stages. Therefore, ZF model could be used as a replacement alternative for water quality testing in order to address one of the long-standing problems of public health concern, ‘Chronic Kidney Disease of unknown origin’ (CKDu) in Sri Lanka.

CKDu is said to be multifactorial in origin leading to hospitalization of over 1,100 CKDu patients per month in Sri Lanka and 300 deaths per year while the first patient was identified in 1994. Total number of patients in Sri Lanka exceeds 70,000. This CKDu problem is prevailing among farming communities and it's a condition, which is slowly progressing and becomes irreversible. Moreover it is asymptomatic until last stages producing mainly tubule-interstitial fibrosis and tubular atrophy as evident in renal biopsies of affected patients [16, 17].

In this context the whole fish as well as its embryo and larvae as per OECD guidelines 236, 203, 210 and 215 could be used to check the effect of suspected heavy metals leading to CKDu and water samples obtained from all sources of water in the endemic areas compared with that of non-endemic areas, as well as with laboratory reconstituted water controls according to the following plan.

1. Collection of water samples from CKDu endemic and non-endemic areas
2. Performance of tests with
    - collected water samples
    - filtered water samples using specially developed filters
    - suspected heavy metals in different concentrations
3. Histopathology with H&E for renal effects using the whole embryo and harvested kidneys of adult fish.

Acknowledgments. I am very thankful to Prof. Hajime Kojima and Prof. Tamaki Yoshikawa for inviting me to share the planned protocol on the use of zebrafish model for CKDu experiments at the Asian congress on alternatives to Animal tests organized by the Japanese society for alternatives to animal experiments. I am grateful to Prof. M A Akbarsha – Director, Mahatma Gandhi– Doerenkamp Center for Alternatives to Use of Animals in Life Science Education, India for recommending me to congress organizers. I also acknowledge the support extended by Prof. Dries Knapen and his team comprising Dr. An Hagenaars, Dr. Lucia Vergauwen and Mrs. Bieke Rutten of University of Antwerp for imparting necessary knowledge and skills related to this model, Dr. Francois Busquet for introducing the author for training at the ZF lab of University of Antwerp, Belgium and the National Science Foundation of Sri Lanka for granting an overseas training fellowship for this purpose.

References

1. Balls M (2009) The three Rs and the humanity criterion: an abridged version of the principles of humane experimental technique by WMS Russell and RL Burch. FRAME, Nottingham, UK
2. Kimmel CB, Ballard WW, Kimmel SR, Ullmann B, and Schilling TF (1995) Stages of embryonic development of the zebrafish. Dev Dyn 203:255–310
3. Nagel R (2000) DarT: the embryo test with the zebrafish danio rerio–a general model in ecotoxicology and toxicology
4. Grunwald DJ, Eisen JS (2002) Headwaters of the zebrafish–emergence of a new model vertebrate. Nar Rev Genet 3:717–724
5. Westerfield M (2007) The zebrafish book, 5th edn: a guide for the laboratory use of zebrafish (Danio rerio). Eugene, University of Oregon Press, USA
6. http://www.hopkinsmedicine.org/news/media/releases/scientists_report_success_using_zebrafish_embryos_to_identify_potential_new_diabetes_drugs. Accessed 27 July 2017

7. Kikuchi K, Poss KD (2012) Cardiac regenerative capacity and mechanisms. Annu Rev Cell Dev Biol 28:719–741
8. Wehner D, Tsarouchas TM, Michael A, Haase C, Weidinger G, Reimer MM, Becker T, Becker CG (2017) Wnt signaling controls pro-regenerative Collagen XII in functional spinal cord regeneration in zebrafish. Nat Commun 8, Article number:126
9. http://www.hopkinsmedicine.org/news/media/releases/immune_system_found_to_control_eye_tissue_renewal_in_zebrafish. Accessed 27 Jul 2017
10. Gunatilake M, Busquet F, Akbarsha MA (2014) Alternatives initiative in Sri Lanka: pre- and post-conference workshops at the inaugural scientific conference of the Sri Lanka association for laboratory animal science. ALTEX 31(2/14):224–226
11. ISO International Organization for Standardization (2007) International standard water quality–determination of the acute toxicity of waste water to zebrafish eggs (Danio Rerio). ISO 15088:2007(E)
12. OECD Publications: OECD guidelines for the testing of chemicals, section 2; effects on biotic systems ISSN: 2074–5761 (online). https://doi.org/10.1787/20745761. www.oecd-ilibrary.org/…/oecd-guidelines-for-the-testing-of-chemicals-section-2-effe. Accessed 17 Jul 2016
13. OECD validation study to assess intra- and inter-laboratory reproducibility of the zebrafish embryo toxicity test for acute aquatic toxicity testing (2014). Busquet et al. Reg Tox and Pharma. http://dx.doi.org/10.1016/j.yrtph.2014.05.018
14. Strahle U, Scholz S, Geisler R, Greiner P, Hollert H, Rastegar S, Schumacher A, Selderslaghs I, Weiss C, Witters H, Braunbeck T (2012) Zebrafish embryos as an alternative to animal experiments-a commentary on the definition of the onset of protected life stages in animal welfare regulations. Reprod Toxicol 33:128–132
15. Dai YJ, Jia YF, Chen N, Bian WP, Li QK, Ma YB, Chen YL, Pei DS (2014) Zebrafish as a model system to study toxicology. Environ Toxicol Chem 33(1):11–7
16. Jayatilake N, Mendis S, Maheepala P, Mehtaet FR (2013) Chronic kidney disease of uncertain aetiology: prevalence and causative factors in a developing country. BMC Nephrol 14:180
17. Redmon JH, Elledge MF, Womack DS, Wickremashinghe R, Wanigasuriya KP, Peiris-John RJ, Lunyera J, Smith K, Raymer JH, Levine KE (2014) Additional perspectives on chronic kidney disease of unknown aetiology (CKDu) in Sri Lanka–lessons learned from the WHO CKDu population prevalence study. BMC Nephrol 15:125

Testing Method Development and Validation for *in Vitro* Skin Irritation Testing (SIT) by Using Reconstructed Human Epidermis (RhE) Skin Equivalent - EPiTRI®

Yu-Chun Lin[1], Hui-Chun Hsu[1], Chiu-Hsing Lin[1], Cheng-Yi Wu[1], Wannhsin Chen[1], and Huey-Min Lai[2](✉)

[1] Biomedical Technology and Device Research Laboratories, Industrial Technology Research Institute (ITRI), Hsinchu TW 300, Taiwan
[2] Biomedical Technology and Device Research Laboratories, Industrial Technology Research Institute (ITRI), Rm 207A Bldg. 13, No. 321, Sect. 2, Kwan-Fu Road, Hsinchu TW 300, Taiwan
HMLai@itri.org.tw

Abstract. Current regulatory requirements focus on assessment of acute irritation potential of chemicals and cosmetics in order to support risk management. A trend has been changed from *in vivo* to *in vitro* testing due to 3R (replacement, reduction, refinement) requirements has resulted from a recent animal testing ban in Taiwan. RhE (Reconstructed human Epidermis) models use normal human keratinocytes to form a multi-layered epidermis including a stratum corneum at the top, which function as a barrier. Some commercialized RhEs passed validation of skin irritation test (SIT) examined by ECVAM, but none of them are originated from Chinese heredity. Therefore, ITRI started a RhE project some years ago based on our long-term developed cell culture experiences, such as isolation of cells from human donors, cell expansion technology, and our own GTP/GMP qualified facilities. So far, a well differentiated and with reproducible barrier function epidermis named EPiTRI® has been reconstructed. We developed a protocol for EPiTRI® SIT in accordance to OECD TG 439. The protocol displays a result of sensitivity of 100%, specificity of 70%, and accuracy of 85% in international validation study. Thus, the human epidermal skin equivalent EPiTRI® can be provided as an *in vitro* model for evaluation of skin irritation and a reliable method has been developed accordingly.

Keywords: Reconstructed human epidermis · Skin irritation test Validation of protocol

Introduction

Topical exposure to chemicals and cosmetic products can lead to various adverse skin effects. Corrosion and irritation are commonly regarded as two major categories among these adverse effects. Corrosive substances irreversibly damage the skin beyond repair, while irritant substances lead to a reversible local inflammatory reaction caused by innate immune system of the affected tissue. Some chemicals trigger an irritant response after

H. Kojima et al. (Eds.): *Alternatives to Animal Testing*, pp. 8–18, 2019.
https://doi.org/10.1007/978-981-13-2447-5_2

repeated exposure to the same skin area, while other chemicals may cause irritation after a single exposure. Current regulatory requirements focus on assessment of acute irritation potential of chemicals and cosmetics in order to support the risk management. Data on skin irritation effects are required by regulatory regimes for chemicals, pesticides, pharmaceuticals and medical devices as a condition of marketing in many countries.

Internationally accepted test methods for skin irritation testing (SIT) include the traditional *in vivo* animal test as well as *in vitro* test methods. However, there is a trend away from *in vivo* to *in vitro* testing due to the 3R (replacement, reduction, refinement) requirement resulted from recent cosmetic animal testing bans in Taiwan and elsewhere. All accepted *in vitro* test methods are based on the RhE technology (Reconstructed human Epidermis) validated by ECVAM. RhE models use normal human keratinocytes which, during culturing, form a multi-layered epidermis including a stratum corneum at the top and can function as a barrier. There are only few RhEs that have been validated for SIT and approved by ECVAM. For the growing Chinese and Asian cosmetic markets, we aimed to develop a human epidermis skin equivalent that contains normal human epidermal structure and function derived from a Chinese population. ITRI has started some years ago in-house based on our culture experience of cells isolated from human donors, the cell expansion (scale up) technology, and our own GTP/GMP facilities. So far, a multi-layered epidermis composed of well differentiated stratified stratum corneum, granulosum, stratum spinosum and basal layer, and with reproducible barrier function, was developed and used for skin irritation testing in accordance to OECD TG 439 guideline.

In this study, we reported the progress about development of reconstructed human epidermis (EPiTRI®) and the aim to develop the skin irritation testing protocol by using EPiTRI® for validation. Quality control parameters for EPiTRI®, such as structure morphology of tissue, thickness, TEER (trans-epithelium electrical resistant), and lipid profile were investigated to study the correlation with barrier function. After obtaining satisfactory quality control data, we conducted the validation process. During protocol development, several important parameters were evaluated for obtaining better statistical accuracy of data when compared with data from *in vivo* testing. These important parameters include pre-incubation time, post-incubation volume, chemical exposure time, washing method, etc. Resulting sensitivity of 100%, specificity of 70% and accuracy of 85% were obtained in current Phase I validation status. The study shows that the human epidermal skin equivalent EPiTRI® could possibly provide as an *in vitro* model to evaluate the skin irritation, and a reliable SIT method has been developed accordingly.

Materials and Methods

EPiTRI® Reconstructed Human Epidermis

EPiTRI® RhE tissue was developed by Biomedical Technology and Device Research Laboratories, ITRI (www.itri.org.tw). The tissue was a three-dimensional and fully differentiated human epidermal skin equivalent, grown from normal human keratinocytes in defined growth medium on the air liquid interface. On day 14, tissues were transferred on nutritive agarose plates and enclosed in a temperature-controlled container for shipment to customers. Each experiment was performed in triplicate on one single tissue production batch, but different batches were used for each repeated experiment. On day 15, EPiTRI® RhE tissues were transferred in 2 mL ITRI culture medium in 6-well plates for an 18–30 h pre-incubation step at 37 ± 1°C, 5 ± 1% CO_2.

Selection of Test Substances

Twenty test substances with diversity of functional chemical groups and physico-chemical properties were selected according to OECD TG 439 (2015) and evaluated by using of EPiTRI®. Details of the 20 test substances are described in Table 2. Phosphate Buffer Saline solution (PBS) treated RhE tissues were used as negative control, Sodium Dodecyl Sulphate (SDS 5% W/V aqueous solution) treated RhE tissues as positive control.

Cell Viability Measurement by MTT Reduction

The MTT (3-[4,5-di-methyl-thiazol-2-yl]-2,5-diphenyl tetrazolium bromide) assay was performed to measure cell viability via converting yellow-colored MTT to blue/purple formazan crystals by dehydrogenases of living cells [3]. Per test conditions, the three EPiTRI® RhE tissues were incubated in 300 μL of MTT solution (1 mg MTT per 1 mL medium) for a 3-h incubation time at 37 ± 1 °C, 5 ± 1% CO_2. Formazan crystal inserts were dissolved in 2 mL isopropanol in 24-well plates for a 3-h extraction time at room temperature.

After extraction, cell viability was analyzed by comparing the optical density of the extracts measured at 570 nm in percentage to the negative PBS treated controls.

In Vitro Skin Irritation Test (SIT)

Step-wised protocol of SIT was shown in Fig. 1. Each test substance was applied topically in triplicate of EPiTRI® RhE tissues. After treatment, tissues were rinsed with PBS and incubated with fresh medium for 42 h at 37 ± 1 °C, 5 ± 1% CO_2. At the end of the incubation, cytotoxicity was determined by MTT conversion test. For each run, the cell viability was calculated and expressed as a percentage relative of the NC. Acceptance criteria for qualified experiment are: (1) $1.0 \leq OD_{570}$ of NC ≤ 2.8; (2) PC $\leq 20\%$; (3) SD of test substance <18%.

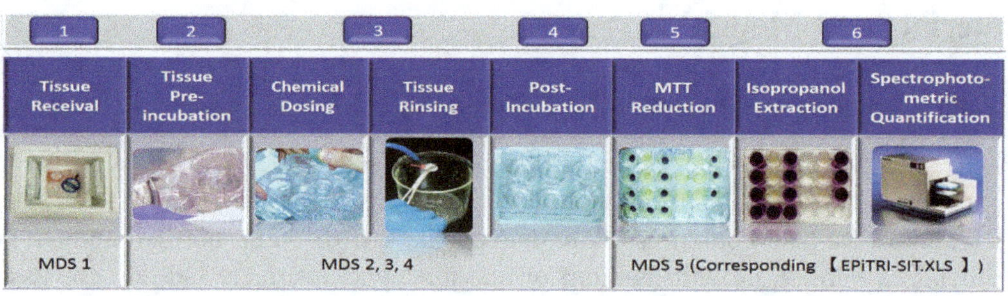

Fig. 1. Protocol of skin irritation test (SIT) developed by ITRI for EPiTRI®

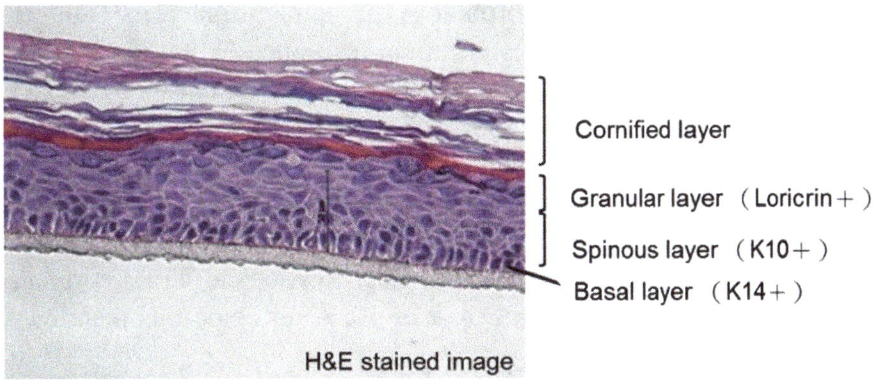

Fig. 2. Structure morphology of EPiTRI® by H&E and immunohistochemical stain

Prediction Model

The SIT protocol allows for prediction of skin irritation potential of test substances according to the United Nations Globally Harmonized System of Classification and Labeling (UN-GHS). Tissue viability that was equal or below 50% of the negative control was used to classify the substance as "Category 2" (Irritant). Tissue viability that was above 50% resulted in classifying the substance as "No category" (Non-irritant).

Statistical Analysis

Mean optical density (OD) and standard deviation (SD) were determined. SD values should be dealt carefully since ECVAM performance standards considers a test as valid only if SD obtained from the three concurrently tested tissues is $\leq 18\%$. The test was evaluated using contingency tables. Sensitivity (percent of Irritant (Category 2) substances correctly predicted *in vitro*), specificity (percent of No category substances correctly predicted *in vitro*) and the concordance (percent of substances correctly classified *in vitro*) were calculated.

Results and Discussions

Change of TER and Structural Morphology during the Reconstruction of EPiTRI®

We have established an efficient protocol in our laboratory for the expansion, differentiation and reconstruction of human skin epidermis equivalent EPiTRI® from primary human keratinocyte. Using our proprietary induction protocol, a multi-layered epidermis composed of stratified stratum corneum, granulosum, stratum spinosum and basal layer were formed after air-lift culture and resembled *in vivo* skin epidermis structure. Moreover, immunohistochemically staining showed that loricrin, cytokeratin 10 and cytokeratin 14 were expressed in the granulosum, spinosum and basal layer respectively, indicating that the reconstructed human epidermis skin equivalent was closely mimic the histology and morphology of human epidermis (Fig. 2). During formation of EPiTRI®, transcutaneous electrical resistance (TER) measurements were performed on EPiTRI® from Day 1 to Day 15. As shown in Fig. 3(A), the TER value was very low at the first three days of differentiation. However, as the epidermis gradually developed, the TER value increased dramatically from Day 3 to Day 9. Process of EPiTRI® differentiation was shown in Fig. 3(B), which displayed a time-coursed maturation of EPiTRI®. As time went by, a multi-layered epidermis was formed. We found that Transcutaneous Electrical Resistance (TER) correlated to the differentiation process from Day 1 to Day 9 or 10. After epidermis matured, the TER maintained at a higher value.

(A)

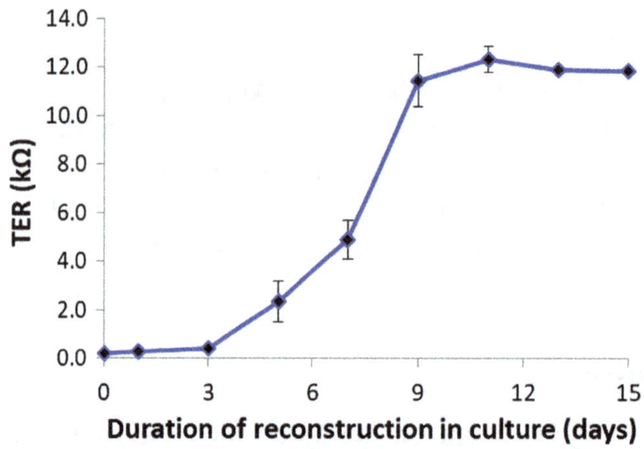

(B)

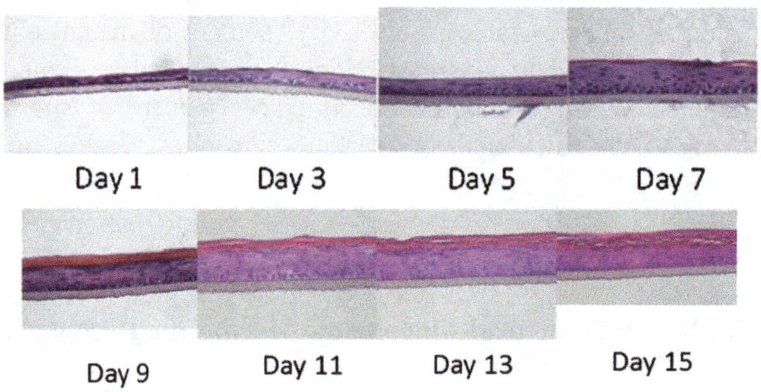

Fig. 3. TER and structural morphology during the reconstruction of EPiTRI®

(A) Transcutaneous electrical resistance (TER) measurements were performed on EPiTRI® from Day1 to Day15. Data represented the average TER of three different tissues at each day point. (B) EPiTRI® skin equivalent shows a time-dependent cell maturation, generating a multi-layer epidermis composed of stratified stratum corneum, granulosum, stratum spinosum and basal layer.

Quality Control of EPiTRI®

In order to meet the requirement of OECD TG 439, the quality control of EPiTRI® is important. Quality factors that we measured include: the thickness of EPiTRI®, the barrier property, the cell viability of negative control and positive control, and transcutaneous electrical resistance. As shown in Fig. 4, the variation on these parameters was small for EPiTRI®. Histology was used to measure the thickness of EPiTRI®. The thickness of EPiTRI® was in the range from 67.06 μm to 85.20 μm (76.32 ± 4.85 μm, CV = 6.36%) (Fig. 4(A)). Negative control OD values of EPITRI® was in the range of 1.33−1.58 (1.44 ± 0.07, CV = 5.2%) (Fig. 4(B)). Measured barrier function of EPiTRI® was in the range of 62.48%−75.01% (70.92 ± 2.53, CV = 4.97%) (Fig. 4(C)). Measurements of TER: 11.3 kΩ−11.9 kΩ (11.6 ± 0.2 kΩ, CV = 1.4%) (Fig. 4(D)).

(A) Thickness of EPiTRI®: 67.06 μm−85.20 μm (76.32 ± 4.85 μm, CV = 6.36%); **(B)** OD values of Negative control: 1.33−1.58 (1.44 ± 0.07, CV = 5.2%); **(C)** Barrier function: of 62.48%−75.01% (70.92 ± 2.53, CV = 4.97%); **(D)** Measurements of TER: 11.3 kΩ−11.9 kΩ (11.6 ± 0.2 kΩ, CV = 1.4%).

Protocol Refinements for the Skin Irritation Test of EPiTRI®

Modification of Washing Method for SIT

Washing method is important in terms of being able to effectively wash away chemicals without damaging the epidermis tissue when considering the development of SIT protocol. We have tried many washing method. Finally, we found an efficient procedure (the last group as shown in Fig. 5(A)) which resulted in the least standard deviation of testing chemicals. Thus we finalized the washing method for SIT in our protocol: Washing off the chemical with continuous stream of PBS at a distance of 3 cm. Squeeze the bottle to maintain a continuous stream of PBS. Then flush the stream against the wall of the insert near the six-o'clock direction for 3 s (4 ± 1 mL). Make sure tissue surface will be fully covered by PBS stream during washing. After washing, discard the PBS into a beaker by taping the insert for three times. Then, gently place the insert on a sterile gauze sponge, tilt the insert on the gauze and tap for three times. Repeat the flushing for another 2 times. Wash off the residual chemical from the insert with PBS for 35 times. To avoid damaging tissues, it is strongly recommended to maintain stable stream of PBS against the wall of the insert.

Chemical Exposure Time

Some parameters in the protocol are critical to develop a successful protocol, for example, chemical exposure time. We found in our experiment for some specific chemicals such as no. 26 and 29, change of exposure time may result in a totally different classification as an irritant or a non-irritant. With 10 min of exposure, they could exhibit non-irritant. However, with 30 min of exposure they apparently are irritant (Fig. 5B).

Pre-incubation Time and Post-incubation Volume

The incubation volume and time are also important to develop a good protocol. Because skin irritation is a reversible reaction, for some chemicals such as No. 19,

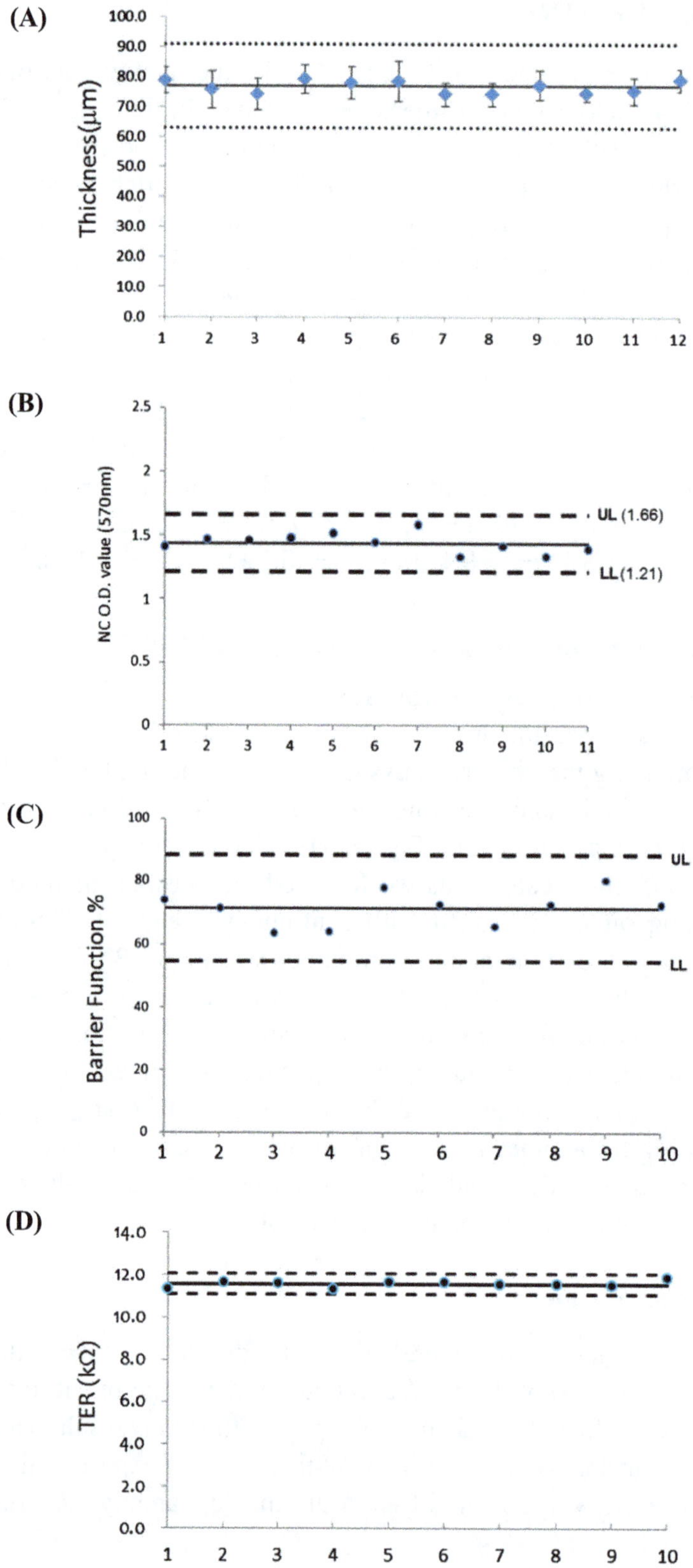

Fig. 4. Quality control of EPiTRI® on **(A)** thickness, **(B)** OD of NC, **(C)** barrier function, and **(D)** TER.

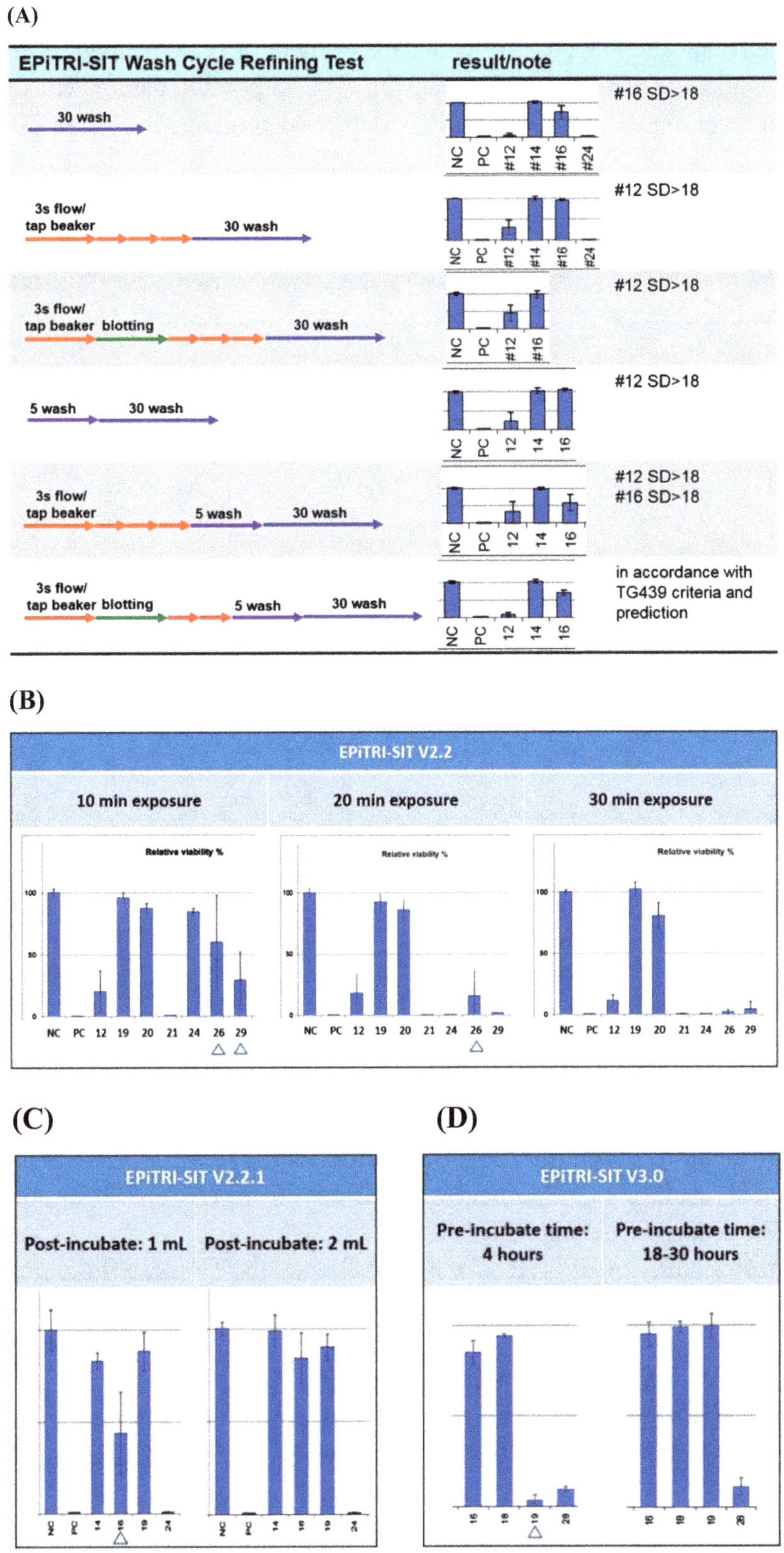

Fig. 5. Protocol refinements for the skin irritation test of EPiTRI®

the increase of pre-incubation time resulted in its classification from irritant to non-irritant. For some chemicals such as No. 16 in our experiment, a post-incubation volume could improve the variation of results (Fig. 5**C, D**). The important parameters of SIT using EPiTRI® when compared with other ECVAM proved products are listed in Table 1.

Table 1. Comparison of EPiTRI®-SIT with validated test tissues in OECD TG 439

Model					
Procedure	EpiSkin™	EpiDerm™ SIT (EPI-200)	SkinEthic™ RHE	LabCyte EPI-MODEL24 SIT	EPiTRI Ver 3.2
Model surface	0.38 cm^2	0.63 cm^2	0.5 cm^2	0.3 cm^2	0.47 cm^2
a) Pre-incubation					
Incubation time	18–24 h	18–24 h	<2 h	15–30 h	18–30 h
Medium volume	2 mL	0.9 mL	0.3 or 1 mL	0.5 mL	2 mL
b) Test chemical application					
For liquids	10 μL (26 μL/cm^2)	30 μL (47 μL/cm^2)	16 μL (32 μL/cm^2)	25 μL (83 μL/cm^2)	35 μL (75 μL/cm^2)
For solids	10 mg (26 mg/cm^2) +DW (5 μL)	25 mg (39 mg/cm^2) +DPBS (25 μL)	16 mg (32 mg/cm^2) +DW (10 μL)	25 mg (83 mg/cm^2) +DW (25 μL)	25 mg (53mg/cm^2) + 20 μL DW
Use of Nylon mesh	not used	if necessary	Applied	not used	S: Applied L: if necessary
Total application time	15 min	60 min	42 min	15 min	30 min
Application temperature	RT	a. RT, 25 min b. 37 °C, 35 min	RT	RT	RT
c) Post-incubation volume					
Medium volume	2 mL	0.9 mL×2	2 mL	1 mL	2 mL
d) Maximum acceptable variability					
SD between tissue replicates	SD ≦ 18	SD ≦ 18	SD ≦ 18	SD ≦ 18	SD ≦ 18

(A) Wash cycle refining test: the last group was selected due to the success of SD < 18 for #12, #14, and #16 chemicals; **(B)** Optimal chemical exposure time was 30 min by using 7 non-coded chemicals. Δ represented SD $\geq$ 18; **(C)** Because the test result of #16 chemical was different from UN GHS Cat. Data exhibited SD $\geq$ 18%, thus 2 mL of medium volume in post-incubation was selected rather than 1 mL; **(D)** Because the test result of #19 chemical was different from UN GHS Cat., thus 18–30 h pre-incubation time was better than 4 h.

In the Phase 1 study of EPiTRI® for SIT, the lead lab ITRI tested the protocol by 20 chemicals (Table 2). Distribution of the testing results of 20 chemicals, with triplicates on each, was shown in Fig. 6 expressed as % cell viability of negative control. 50% viability cut-off was used for the prediction of irritants and non-irritants. The predictive capacity in terms of sensitivity, specificity and accuracy, we obtained scores of 100%, 70%, and 85%, respectively (Table 3). Meet the requirement of OECD TG 439.

Three independent experiments performed for each reference chemical. Distribution of the 20 chemical test results, the average of the three experiments for each data point, shown as % of tissue viability of negative control. 50% viability cut-off was used for the prediction of irritants from non-irritants.

Table 2. Twenty selected test substances and predictive capacity of EPiTRI® in comparison with GHS Category or OECD VRM

Test substances	CAS No.	Storage	Physical state	VRM Cat. based on in vitro	UN GHS Cat. based on in vivo results	In vivo score
l-bromo-4-chlorobutane	6940-78-9	RT	Liquid	Cat. 2	No Cat.	0
Diethyl phthalate	84-66-2	RT	Liquid	No Cat.	No Cat.	0
Naphthalene acetic acid	86-87-3	RT	Solid	No Cat.	No Cat.	0
Allyl phenoxy-acetate	7493-74-5	RT	Liquid	No Cat.	No Cat.	0.3
Isopropanol	67-63-0	RT	Liquid	No Cat.	No Cat.	0.3
4-{methylthio)-benzaldehyde	3446-89-7	RT	Liquid	Cat. 2	No Cat.	1
Methyl stearate	112-61-8	-20 °C	Solid	No Cat.	No Cat.	1
Heptyl butyrate	5870-93-9	RT	Liquid	No Cat.	NoCat.(Optional Cat. 3)	1.7
Hexyl salicylate	6259-76-3	RT	Liquid	No Cat.	NoCat.(Optional Cat. 3)	2
Cinnamaldehyde	104-55-2	4 °C	Liquid	Cat. 2	No Cat.(Optional Cat. 3)	2
1-decanol	112-30-1	RT	Liquid	Cat. 2	Cat. 2	2.3
Cyclamen aldehyde	103-95-7	RT	Liquid	Cat. 2	Cat. 2	2.3
1-bromohexane	111-25-1	RT	Liquid	Cat. 2	Cat. 2	2.7
2-chloromethyl-3,S-dimethyl-4- methoxypyridine HCI	86604-75-3	RT	Solid	Cat. 2	Cat. 2	2.7
Di-n-propyl disulphide	629-19-6	RT	Liquid	No Cat.	Cat. 2	3
Potassium hydroxide (5% aq.)	1310-58-3	RT	Liquid	Cat. 2	Cat. 2	3
Benzenethiol, 5 (1,1-dimethylethyl)-2-methyl	7340-90-1	RT	Liquid	Cat. 2	Cat. 2	3.3
l-methyl-3-phenyl-l-piperazine	5271-27-2	RT	Solid	Cat. 2	Cat. 2	3.3
Heptanal	111-71-7	RT	Liquid	Cat. 2	Cat. 2	3.4
Tetrachloroethylene	127-18-4	RT	Liquid	Cat. 2	Cat. 2	4

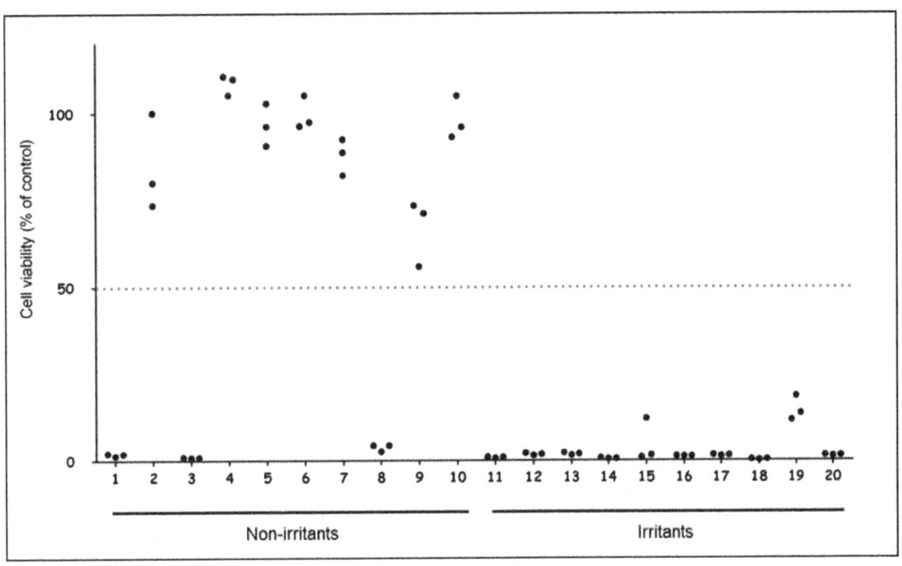

Fig. 6. Distribution of the relative tissue viability obtained with the treatment of 20 selected chemical substances on EPiTRI®.

Table 3. The predictive capacity recommended by OECD TG 439 and tested result on EPiTRI®

Predictive capacity	OECD TG439 recommendation (%)	EPiTRI-SIT
Sensitivity	80%	100%(10/10)
Specificity	70%	70% (7/10)
Accuracy	75%	85% (17/20)

Conclusion

In this study, the good quality of RhE (EPiTRI®) model was presented in terms of its stable thickness, TER, structural morphology and barrier function. Furthermore, we demonstrated the development of a reliable SIT protocol using of EPiTRI®, producing an overall sensitivity of 100%, specificity of 70% and accuracy of 85%. These results meet the OECD guidelines. Based on its high predictive capacity, our *in vitro* SIT with EPiTRI® could be a promising alternative to *in vivo* SIT.

References

1. Protocol of *In Vitro* Skin Irritation: Human Epidermis Model: EPiTRI®-SIT V3.2
2. OECD Guidelines for the Testing of Chemicals (2015), *In Vitro* Skin Irritation: Reconstructed Human Epidermis Test Method
3. Mosmann T (1983) Rapid colorimetric assay for cellular growth and survival: application to proliferation and cytotoxicity assays. J Immunol Methods 65:55–63
4. Frank N (2005) The human epidermis models EpiSkin, SkinEthic and EpiDerm: an evaluation of morphology and their suitability for testing phototoxicity, irritancy, corrosivity, and substance transport. Eur J Pharm Biopharm 60:167–178
5. Carine T (2006) *In vitro* skin irritation testing on reconstituted human epidermis: reproducibility for 50 chemicals tested with two protocols. Toxicol in Vitro 20:401–416
6. Martin M (2009) A tiered approach to the use of alternatives to animal testing for the safety assessment of cosmetics: skin irritation. Regul Toxicol Pharmacol 54:188–196
7. Carine T (2010) Assessment of the optimized SkinEthic™ Reconstructed Human Epidermis (RHE) 42 bis skin irritation protocol over 39 test substances. Toxicol in Vitro 24:245–256
8. Masakazu K (2011) Refinement of LabCyte EPI-MODEL24 skin Irritation test method for adaptation to the requirements of OECD test guideline TG 439. Altern Anim Test Exp 16:111–122
9. Hajime K (2013) A catch-up validation study of an *in vitro* skin irritation test method using reconstructed human epidermis LabCyte EPI-MODEL24. J Appl Toxicol 34:766–774

Development the Technique for the Preparation and Characterization of Reconstructed Human Epidermis (RHE)

Herlina B. Setijanti[1,2], Eka Rusmawati[1(✉)], Rahmi Fitria[1], Tuty Erlina[1], Rina Adriany[1], and Murtiningsih[1]

[1] Research Centre for Drug and Food, National Agency Drug and Food Control of Republic of Indonesia, Central Jakarta, Indonesia
bs_herlina_2002@yahoo.com
[2] Faculty of Pharmacy and Science, HAMKA University of Republic of Indonesia, South Jakarta, Indonesia

Abstract. Reconstructed Human Epidermis (RHE) is an artificial epidermis made in such a way that it resembles human skin, and can be used for the identification of irritant chemicals, especially for cosmetic and topical medicinal products. Currently the new RHE is produced by European and American countries, whose skin physiology is very different from Indonesia. Based on this, the Center for Research on Drugs and Food, NADFC of Republic of Indonesia took the initiative to develop the reconstruction of keratinocyte, melanocytes and fibroblasts cells into RHE adapted to the anatomical and physiological functions of the skin of Indonesians. RHE is made from an epidermal layer composed of keratinocyte and melanocytes cells that are reconstructed with a dermis layer composed of fibroblast and collagen cells. Keratinocyte, melanocytes and fibroblasts cells are cultured on suitable mediums by adding a suitable growth medium. To find out that RHE has been successfully reconstructed, measured percentage of cell life, made histology preparation to see the existence of cell nucleus, and conducted Immunohistochemical examination to see existence of integration (bond) between antigen. From the research results can be seen that keratinocyte cells grown on culture medium Keratinocyte SFM (IX) with rEGF supplements; melanocyte cells grown on Melanocyte 254 culture medium with HMGS supplementation; and fibroblast cells grown on Fibroblast M 106 culture medium with LSGS supplementation. The percentage of epidermal cell life grew well in the planting of 10×10^4 cells /mL keratinocytes and 0.25×10^4 cells /mL of melanocyte cells and survived until the 11th day with live cell percentage of 93.45%. In making preparation for histology with HE staining, there is a cell life in RHE tissue. Used Immunohistochemical (IHC) examination using cytokeratin 10 antibody marker to view physiological function of epidermal tissue.

Keywords: RHE · Keratinocytes cell · Melanocyte cell

H. Kojima et al. (Eds.): *Alternatives to Animal Testing*, pp. 20–32, 2019.
https://doi.org/10.1007/978-981-13-2447-5_3

Back Ground

The wide use of cosmetics and the many types of cosmetics circulating in Indonesia need strict supervision by the National Agency of Drug and Food Control (NADFC) to ensure its safety and do not cause irritation and allergies.

Testing irritation and allergies on the skin previously carried out by using rabbits and albino guinea pig, but with the widespread animal welfare issues causing restrictions on the use of experimental animals. So it is necessary to develop the method of skin irritation test in vitro, one of them by using Reconstructed Human Epidermis or RHE (Nelson et al. 1980).

RHE is an artificial epidermis made in such a way that its anatomy and physiology resemble human skin, and can be used for the identification of irritant chemicals, especially for cosmetic products and medical devices (Rehder 2004). Currently RHE is newly produced by European and American countries, whose skin physiology is very different from Indonesian skin physiology, so that RHE production in Indonesia is considered very important, economical in terms of production, and reduce dependence on other countries. Other advantages of in vitro toxicity testing are easy to do, efficient and economical.

Structure of Skin Networks

The skin is the largest organ of the body and has two major layers, the epidermis and the dermis. Each of these layers has specific functions and structures. The skin tissue structure can be described as Fig. 1.

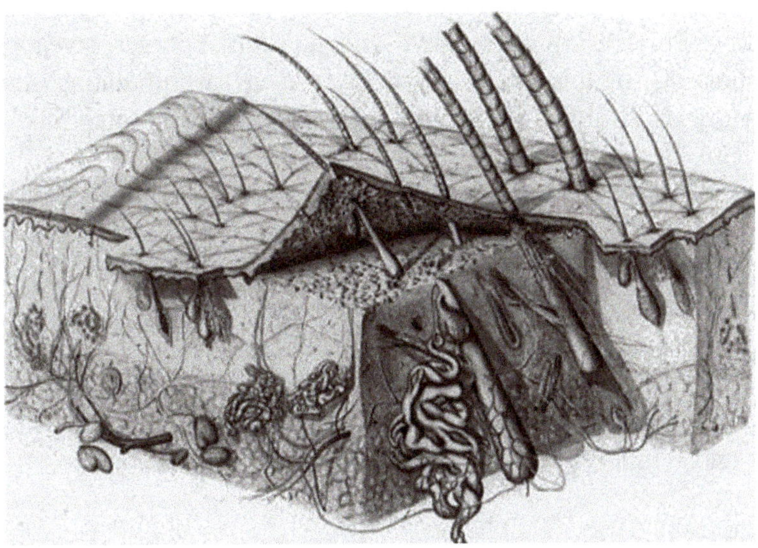

Fig. 1. Diagram of the structure of human skin tissue

The epidermis occupies the outermost layer, followed by the dermis layer and the hypodermic. The epidermis is an elastic layer and continues to be regenerated, whereas the dermis is the inner layer that includes the sweat glands and produces sweat that travels through the sweat channel to the pores that play a role in temperature regulation. In the layers below the dermis there is a hypodermis composed of fatty tissue or adipose tissue where there are many veins and arteries located between the dermis and hypodermic layers (Montagna 1974).

Epidermis

The skin epidermis layer consists of the horn layer or corneum layer and the Malpighi layer. The horn or corneum layer is a layer of dead skin, which can be peeled off and replaced by new cells, while the Malpighi layer consists of layers of spinosum and germinativum, each of which has its own function. In addition, the epidermal skin layer contains a melanin pigment that gives color to the skin, therefore it is important to keep the skin from UV radiation that can burn the skin and change the color of the skin becomes darker.

The epidermis is the outermost layer of the human skin and consists of layers such as: melanocytes that produce melanin, langerhans cells which has an important role in skin immunology, and Merkel cells that act as sensory mechanoreceptor. Keratinocytes layer composed of several stratums are the Stratum korneum, Stratum lucidum, Stratum granulosum, Stratum spinosum, Stratum Basal, which is the lowest layer of the epidermis (Schallreuter and dan Wood 1995).

Dermis

The dermis skin layer consists of blood vessels, hair roots, nerves, sweat glands and oil glands. The function of this dermis skin layer is as a stimulating receptor organ, protective against physical damage, illumination and disease protection, as well as for regulation of body temperature.

The dermis skin layer is at the bottom of the epidermis skin which has two stratum structures, namely the Stratum papilare which contain fibroblasts and stratum reticular which composed of connective tissue (especially type 1 collagen). In addition to these two stratum the dermis also contains some epidermal derivatives namely hair follicles, sweat glands, and sebaceous glands. Below the dermis there is a layer of loose connective tissue called the subcutaneous tissue and contains fat cells. This network is also called superficial fascia or paniculus adiposus. This tissue contains rich bundles of blood vessels and lymph vessels (Montagna 1974).

Keratinocytes Cells

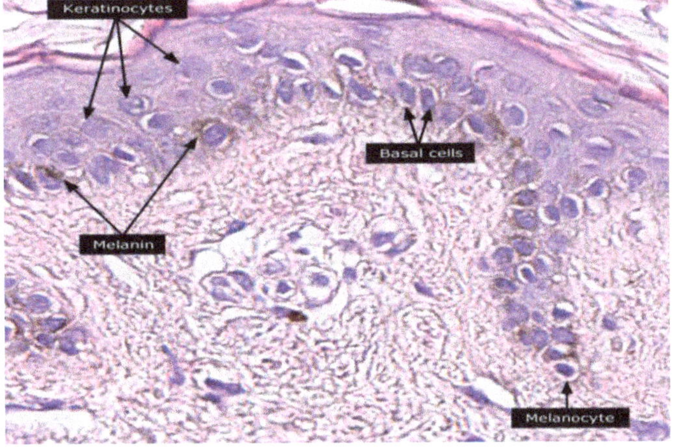

Fig. 2. Skin epidermis with keratinocyte and melanocytes cells

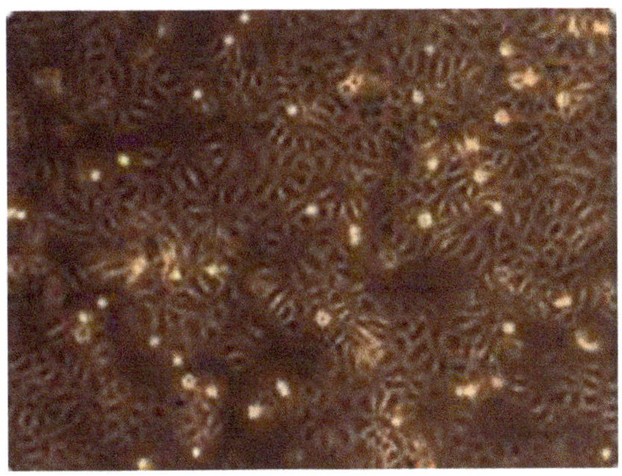

Fig. 3. Keratinocyte cells on day 5 in the media culture

Keratinocytes are a type of cell that dominates 90% more cells that exist in the outermost layer of the skin (epidermis). Keratinocytes are found in the basal layer (Stratum germinativum) of the skin to be referred to as "basal cells" or "basal keratinocytes". Squamous keratinocytes are found in the oral and esophageal mucosa, as well as the cornea, conjunctiva, and genital epithelium (Morgan 2003) (Figs. 2 and 3).

The main function of keratinocytes is as a barrier to environmental damage such as pathogen bacteria or fungi or viruses, heat, UV radiation and water loss. When pathogen invade the epidermal top layer, keratinocytes may react by producing certain proinflammatory and chemokine mediators such as interleukin 1, interleukin 2, interleukin 6, and TNF-α that attract leukocytes to site of pathogen invasion (Morgan 2003).

A number of structural proteins (filaggrin, keratin), enzymes (proteases), lipids and antimicrobial peptides (defensin) contribute to maintaining important skin barrier functions. Keratinization is part of the formation of a physical barrier (cornification), in which keratinocytes produce keratin as an overriding primary protein and eventually undergo programmed cell death. Keratin is what makes up the hair and nails (Morgan 2003).

Melanocytes Cell

Melanocytes are somatic cells that produce melanin, providing important physiological functions in the epidermal basal layer (stratum basal) of the skin, the middle layer of the eye (uvea), the inner ear, the bone, and the liver. Functions related to human melanin production include photo protection, capture of reactive oxygen, execution of metal ions, and bind to certain drugs and organic chemicals (Tolleson 2005). Melanin is the main pigment responsible for skin color. Melanin is dark and absorbs all UV-B light. This melanin is produced through a process called melanogenesis. This melanogenesis

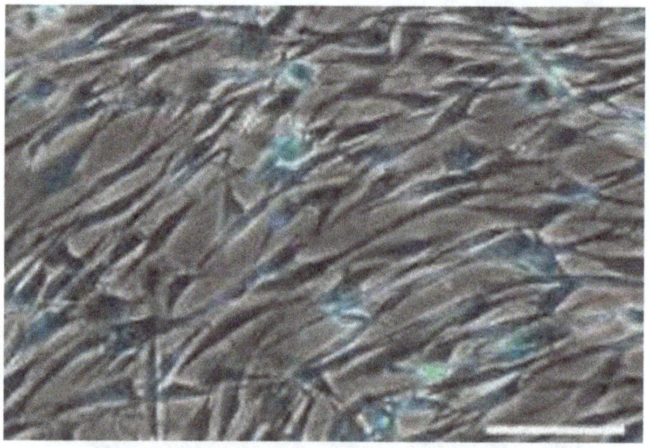

Fig. 4. Melanocyte cell on day 3 in culture medium M 254

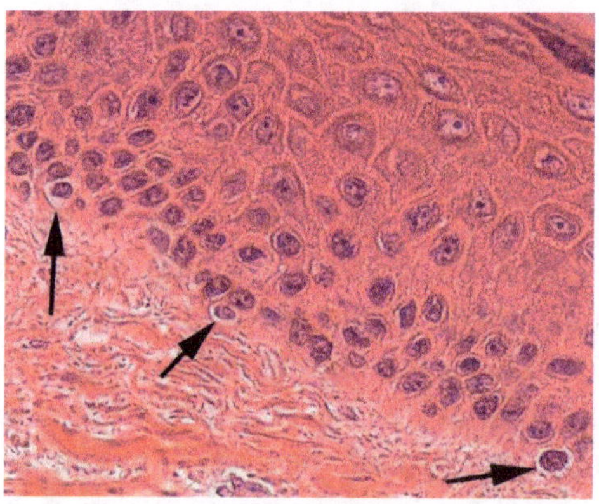

Fig. 5. Melanocyte cells in the epidermal tissue of human skin

causes pigmentation, which is different from the pigmentation derived from the existing melanin oxidation. In general, lighter-skinned people have low-grade basal melanogenesis. Exposure to UV-B radiation causes melanogenesis to increase. The goal of melanogenesis is to protect the hypodermis, the lower layers of the skin, from UV-B rays that can damage DNA (Tolleson 2005) (Figs. 4 and 5).

In general, for per square millimeter of skin containing between 1000 and 2000 melanocytes. The difference in skin color between light and dark of a pigmented individual is due to the amount of melanocytes in their skin, but to the extent of melanocyte activity depends greatly on the quantity and relative amount of eumelanin and pheomelanin). This process is under hormonal control, including peptides from Melanocyte-Stimulating Hormones (MSH) and Adrenocorticotropic Hormone (ACTH) resulting from propiomelanocortin precursor.

Fibroblasts Cell

Fibroblasts are cells that produce collagen and elastin that provide a middle layer of skin structure called the dermis. The dermis is the middle layer of the skin (below the epidermis) containing collagen fibers, elastic fibers, hyaluronic acid, blood vessels and lymphatic vessels, hair follicles, nerves, glands, and many others. This dermis is the "brain" of the skin, also called kutis (Doyle and dan Griffiths 2000).

Fibroblast cells include connective tissue because fibroblast cells have an important role in the formation of connective tissue that is forming fibers (collagen, reticular, and elastin) and producing macromolecules (glycosaminoglycans and proteoglycans) which are the basic components of connective tissue, because the cells are relatively stable and very little of movement.

Elastin is a structural protein that forms thin elastic fibers, similar to collagen. This material is produced by fibroblasts and serves to restore the skin to its position while

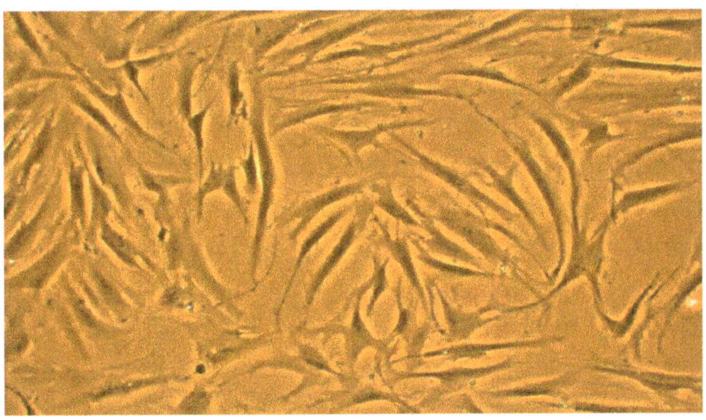

Fig. 6. Fibroblast cells in culture medium containing FBS with 10x magnification

resting. Collagen is a protein that is a major element of connective tissue and bone, and provides strength and endurance to the skin. Aging causes a decrease in collagen production that causes thinning, wrinkled, and sagging skin. Collagen in skin cream is almost useless, but collagen can be stimulated with retinoids, vitamin C and some other antioxidants, lasers and certain injections (Harlystiarini 2010) (Fig. 6).

Reconstruct Ed Human Epiderm is (Rhe)

Reconstructed Human Epidermis (RHE) is defined as human skin tissue obtained from the in vitro process in which human keratinocyte cells are cultured on an inert polycarbonate medium. RHE has a major advantage for growing donor epidermal cells in a serum-free culture environment. After the preparation of the acquired keratinocyte culture has rapidly multiplied, the epidermal cells produced on the inert filter substrate are lifted to the air-fluid interface in the CO_2 incubator. A nutrient medium as a food of the basal cells through sub-stratum filters. After 14 days, a stratified epidermis has formed that resembles the human epidermis in vivo. Morphologically, this culture shows stratified epithelial and cornified epidermis by significantly improving barrier function and metabolic activity. Marker differentiation such as keratin suprabasal, integrin b4, integrin a6, fibronectin, involucrin, filaggrin, trichohyalin, type I, III, IV, V and VII collagen, laminin, heparin sulfate and membrane-bound transglutaminase have been found, presented similarly to human epidermis (Rehder 2004).

RHE is formed from a layer of an inert filter substrate containing collagen with fibroblast cells and cultured in an appropriate medium. This layer is a feeder layer that will become the growth medium of keratinocyte cells and melanocytes as the composer of the artificial skin epidermis. RHE can also be composed of keratinocyte cells and melanocytes cultured on biological matrix and the system stored at the air-liquid interface, in a suitable culture medium, to form a human epidermal layer with histologic characteristics of the epidermis in vivo. RHE is considered good when histologic observations indicate reconstructed in vitro epidermis has a similar arrangement of human epidermis in the correct position, with functional keratinocytes and melanocytes similar to in vivo epidermis (Rehder 2004).

The function of RHE is very important as an alternate model of animal experiments for testing the toxicity and effects of topical products since current testing of cosmetic products with experimental animals has been prohibited. In vitro testing using the reconstructed human skin epidermal tissue model (RHE) has been widely used in the cosmetics, pharmaceutical and chemical industries as an alternative to animal testing for various applications including toxicity, efficacy, pharmacology and skin absorption studies. The pharmaceutical and dermocosmetic industries have switched to using the human skin epidermis that was reconstructed into RHE as a model for testing such as: skin penetration rates of various substances, inflammatory reactions, effects of ultraviolet radiation, hormone metabolism and so on. The continuous improvement of this model makes an efficient predictor for research and development of topical toxicity tests (Nelson et al. 1980).

Various Models for epidermal testing have passed scientific validation in ECVAM (European Committee Validation of Alternative Method, a Validation Center for Alternative Methods for European Veterinary Testing) to predict skin irritation and be accepted for regulatory purposes in predicting skin corrosion (OECD 2013) and skin permeation (OECD 2004). But now all models have been properly validated, protected by patents and/or are traded using proprietary tissue culture procedures by some private companies, so its availability depends entirely on the strategy of each company (Berking and dan Herlyn 2001).

The epidermis of the skin is an important tissue that produces a strong internal organ body protector, flexible and able to repair itself against environmental influences. Its main function is to protect the body from dehydration, loss of nutrients and unwanted effects due to substances that contact with the skin in various forms depending on its physicochemical properties. The epidermis can contribute to the protection of living organisms that we encounter around us, such as animals, plants and fungi, as well as invisible micro-organisms by the human eye such as bacteria and viruses.

In order to be and remain effective, the epidermal layer should be able to protect the body from the substance most often potentially harmful to physical, chemical or biological. Therefore, most epidermal studies are related to the production, maintenance and repair of the epidermal layer (Poumay and dan Coquette 2007). Since the skin is often exposed to cosmetic products or other ingredients whether intentionally or not, the potential for irritation or corrosion of the skin is large enough that as part of the overall safety assessment process, a product must be carefully evaluated.

Skin Irritation Test

Skin irritation test can be done both in vivo and in vitro. In vivo testing typically used experimental animals as albino rabbits, while in vitro testing was used as an experimental model of RHE. In vitro testing is a strategy for assessing potential corrosion and irritation. Testing of chemicals for skin irritation after acute exposure is considered to be one way to evaluate the toxicology of simple endpoints. Historically, this process involves only exposure to chemicals in rabbit skin and observing the results (OECD 2010). Over the past decade, various non-animal test methods (in vitro tests) have been developed and validated to predict the potential for skin corrosion and chemical skin irritation (Doucet et al. 2010).

Examination of Histology Network with Hematoxyline - Eosin Determination

Histology is a branch of biological science that studies the structure of tissues in detail using a microscope on a thinly cut tissue preparation. Histology can also be referred to as a microscopic anatomical science.

Histology is divided into two parts: general histology that includes studies of tissues contained in the body and special histology or organ histology that includes the histological structure of the organs of the body. The tissues of the body are formed by two interacting components of the cell and the extracellular matrix. The extracellular matrix consists of many types of molecules, and most of them are very complex and form complex structures, such as fibers and basement membranes. To analyze the tissue structure that has been cut thinly used the method of haematoxylin-eosin staining (HE), because this coloration can show most of the histology structure. The hematoxillin will form the nucleus of the cell (nucleus) and other acidic structures of the cell (such as the RNA-rich portion of the cytoplasm and the cartilage matrix) into blue, while the Eosin is acidic, which will color the cytoplasm and collagen into pink (Dharma 1985).

Immunohistochemical (IHC)

Immunohistochemistry is a method to detect proteins in cells of a tissue by using the principle of binding between antibodies and antigens in living tissues. Immunohistochemical painting are widely used in the examination of abnormal cells such as cancer cells. Specific molecules will color certain cells such as dividing cells or dead cells that can be distinguished from normal cells. This check requires a network.

of varying amounts and thicknesses depending on the purpose of the inspection. Generally the tissues that come from the body will be cut into very thin pieces by using a tool called vibrating microtome.

Some commonly used immunohistochemical examples include Keratin 10, Carcino Embryonic Antigen (CEA), CD 15, CD 30, Prostate Spesific Antigen (PSA), CD 117, Estrogen and Progesteron, CD 20 and CD 3.

Result and Discussion

Cell Culture of Keratinocytes, Melanocytes and Fibroblasts

Keratinocyte cells in culture using Keratinocyte SFM (IX) medium, with addition of human recombinant Epidermal Growth Factor (rEGF) and Bovine Pituitary Extract (BPE). The 7th day keratinocytes and confluent 11th day keratinocytes can be observed with an inverted microscope of 100 × magnification.

Melanocyte cells in culture using 254 Medium plus Human Melanocyte Growth Supplement (HMGS). The 3rd day melanocytes and confluent 6th day of melanocyte can be observed with an inverted microscope of 100 × magnification.

Fibroblast cells in culture using M 106 Medium plus LSGS supplement. The 4th day fibroblast cells and confluent 7th day of fibroblast can be observed with an inverted microscope of 100 × magnification.

Making of Feeder Layer (Dermis Eqivalen)

The feeder layer (dermis eqivalen) is made of a mixture of fibroblasts and collagen cells that function as a scaffold in the preparation of RHE. The results show that the eqivalent dermis forms a layer that does not stick to the bottom of the plate, can be observed after incubation for 3 days at 37 °C using 5% CO_2 incubator.

Making of RHE Tissue (Reconstructed Human Epidermis)

The RHE is made of from the eqivalent dermis layer coated with the epidermis layer,

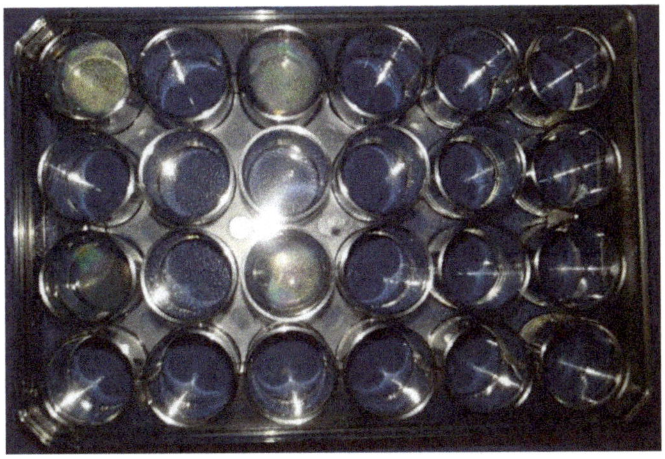

Fig. 7. RHE tissue consisting of an equivalent dermis and epidermal layer

where the epidermis layer is on the seedling above the sterile insert comprising a mixture of keratinocyte cells and melanocyte cells in ratio (40: 1), then cultured on an epidermal medium (IMDM) containing vitamin C 37.5 μg/mL. The purpose of adding vitamin C to the culture medium is as an antioxidant to strengthen the epidermal membrane layer so that the layer is not easily separated. The results of making RHE network can be seen in Fig. 7.

Measuring of Cell Life Using MTT Method

Measurements of cell life from RHE tissue were used MTT method, wherein keratinocyte and melanocyte cell life was obtained by calculation using formula:

$$\% \text{ celllife} = \frac{\text{treatmentabsorption} - \text{blankoabsorption} \times 100\%\text{Blankoabsorption}}{\text{Blankoabsorption}}$$

Measurements of cell life from the epidermal layer were performed on day 1 (considered as base line), day 3, day 7, day 11 and day 14. The increase in the number of living cells occurred only until the 7th day, then there was a decrease on the 11th day. This may be due to the fact that the number of keratinocyte and melanocyte cells grown too much, so that the availability of culture media on the propylene ring is insufficient, eventually the growth of cells in the tissue becomes blocked and some die.

Epidermis layer production is repeated by decreasing the number of planting cells to one fifth of the number of cells grown in the first experiment. So the number of cells changed from 50 × 104 cell/mL to 10 × 104 cell/mL for keratinocyte cells and 1,25 × 104 cell/mL to 0,25 × 104 cell/mL for melanocyte cells.

Making Histology Preparations of Reconstructed Human Epiderm Using Staining of Hematoxylin-Eosin (HE)

Hematoxylin and Eosin are coloring methods that are widely used in the staining of histological tissues. Hematoxylin memulas the nucleus and other acidic structures of

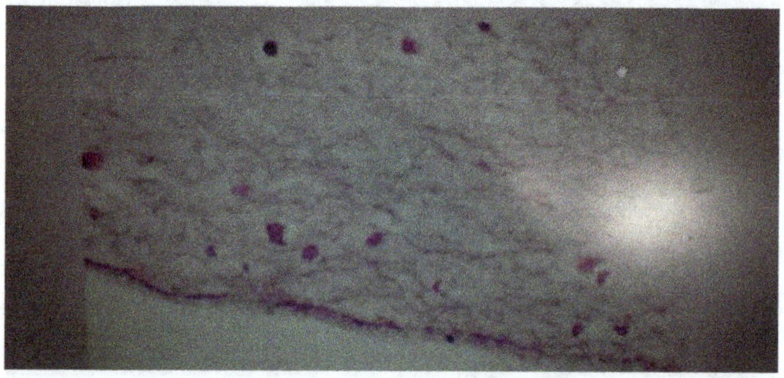

Fig. 8. The results of skin tissue reconstruction on the 11th day

the cell (such as the RNA-rich cytoplasm section and cartilage matrix) to blue/purple. Haematoxylin will color the nucleus while eosin will color the cytoplasm. Eosin is acidic, which will color the cytoplasm and collagen into pink.

The result of preparation of histology and staining using HE can be seen in Fig. 8 here is the presence of cell nucleus (purple blue color) but not yet showing the formation of tissue component (not yet showing any protein expressed in skin tissue), so immunohistochemistry is needed antibody (marker) that is specific to skin tissue.

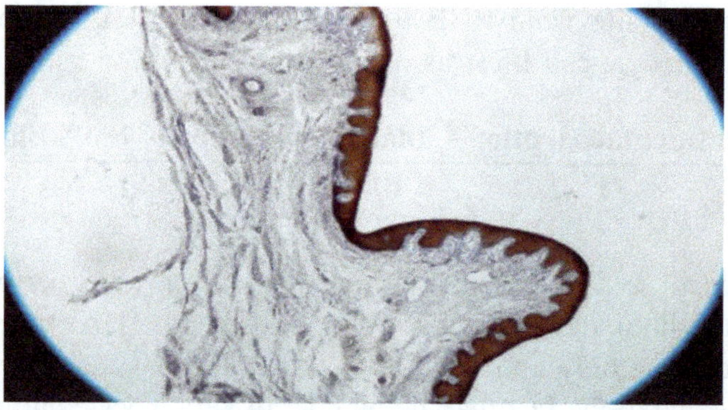

Fig. 9. IHC examination of normal skin tissue

Immunohistochemical (IHC) Examination of RHE Skin Tissue Using Cytokeratin 10 Antibody Marker

Immunohistochemical (IHC) is a technique for detecting a specific protein (antigen) in tissues or cells using specific antibodies (markers). The purpose of this IHC examination is to validate the reconstructed skin tissue, using antibodies specific to the epidermis. The results of immunohistochemical examination of RHE skin tissue can be seen in Fig. 9.

The results of IHC examination of reconstructed skin tissue using cytokeratin 10 antibody marker have not shown any integration (bonding) between the epidermal layer with the marker, this is probably because the proteins formed are incompatible with antibody cytokeratin 10. Other possibilities is not yet formed protein so physiological function of the epidermis has not existed, therefore RHE skin tissue cannot be used as skin irritation test model in vitro.

Conclusion

Keratinocyte, melanocytes and fibroblasts cells can grow well on suitable medium with the addition of suitable growth medium that is keratinocyte cells grown on Keratinocyte SFM (IX) culture medium with Human recombinant supplement (rEGF); melanocyte cells grown on Melanocyte 254 culture medium with HMGS.

supplementation; and fibroblast cells grown on Fibroblast M 106 culture medium with LSGS supplementation. The percentage of epidermal cell life grew well in the planting of 10 × 104 cells /mL keratinocytes and 0.25 × 104 cells /mL of melanocyte cells and survived until the 11th day with live cell percentage of 93.45%. The preparation of histology preparations with HE staining shows the presence of cell life in RHE tissue. IHC examination using cytokeratin 10 antibody marker not shows any physiological function of the epidermis tissue.

References

Berking C, dan Herlyn M (2001) Human skin reconstruct models: a new applicationfor studies of melanocyte and melanoma. Biology Histol Histopathol 16:669–674

Dharma A (1985) Basic Histology

Doucet O et al (2010) A catch-up validation study on reconstructed human epidermis (SkinEthicTM RHE) for full replacement of the Draize skin irritation test, Toxicology in Vitro, 257–266

Doyle A, dan Griffiths JB (2000) Cell and tissue culture for medical research. John Willey & Sons Ltd, England

Harlystiarini (2010) In Vitro Fibroblast in culture. Bogor Agriculture University

Montagna W (1974) The structure and function of skin. Academy Press, New York, London

Morgan GA (2003) Experimental model of cultured keratinocytes. Acta Cir Bras [serial online], vol 18 Special Edition

Nelson PH et al (1980) Optimized condition for the growth of human epidermis cell in culture. J Investig Dermatol 75:176–182

OECD (2004) *Guideline* For The Testing Of Chemicals. In Vitro Skin Irritation Reconstructed Human Epidermis Test Method, Test No, p 428

OECD (2010) Guideline for the testing of chemicals. In Vitro skin irritation reconstructed human epidermis test method, Test No. 439

OECD (2013) Guideline for the testing of chemicals. In Vitro skin corrosion: reconstructed human epidermis (RHE) Test method Test No. 431

Poumay Y, dan Coquette A (2007) Modelling the human epidermis in vitro: tools for basic and applied research. Arch Dermatol Res 298:361–369

Rehder J et al (2004) Model of human epidermis reconstructed in vitro with keratinocytes and melanocytes on dead de-epidermized human dermis. Sao Paulo Med J 122(1):22–25

Schallreuter KU, dan Wood JM (1995) The human epidermis. Proc Nutrition Soc 54:191–195

Tolleson WH (2005) Human melanocyte biology. Toxicol Pathol J Environ Sci Health 23:105–161

Alternative Research (3Rs) in the World, Asia and Japan

Tsutomu Miki Kurosawa(✉)

Joint Faculty of Veterinary Medicine, Kagoshima University, Kagoshima, Japan
japanawrl@gmail.com

Alternative research is currently conducted all over the world and its recent progress is remarkable as 3Rs research. This article describes a review of alternative research and 3Rs in the world, Asia and Japan.

The World

"Principles of Humane Experimental Technique" were first articulated in the 1950s by Russell and Burch (1959), giving birth to a new field of laboratory animal welfare and the "3Rs" concept of replacement, reduction and refinement in life sciences research. A decade later, the Fund for the Replacement of Animals in Medical Experiments (FRAME 2018) was founded, with a mission to support alternative research, together with the journal Alternatives to Laboratory Animals (ATLA), which has become a leading academic journal of this field.

In 1981, the Center for Alternatives to Animal Testing (CAAT) was founded at Johns Hopkins University. The center co-organized the 1st World Congress on Alternatives and Animal Use in the Life Sciences in 1993 (CAAT 2018). The first president of World Congress of Alternatives was Dr. Alan Goldberg and then he is one of the prominent leaders of this field. His remarkable effort of alternatives to animal testing in toxicology is realistic strategy for alternative research. Because the most of chemicals should be tested their safety before marketing, the toxicological study using animals was a common sense in this field. However, Dr. Goldberg proposes many non-animal testing methods for their safety.

The European Reference Laboratory for Alternatives to Animal Testing (EURL-ECVAM) (ECVAM 2018), founded in 1991 as the European Centre for the Validation of Alternative Methods, was given a new name and broader mandate in 2010 for promoting the not only scientific but also regulatory acceptance of non-animal tests which are of importance to biomedical sciences. EURL-ECVAM does so by supporting research, test development and validation, the establishment of a specialised database service, and engagement with international academic organizations in this field. Their targets include chemicals and products of various kinds, including medicines, vaccines, medical devices, cosmetics, household products and agricultural products.

H. Kojima et al. (Eds.): *Alternatives to Animal Testing*, pp. 33–36, 2019.
https://doi.org/10.1007/978-981-13-2447-5_4

The US Interagency Coordinating Committee on the Validation of Alternative Methods (ICCVAM) was established by law in 2000 (ICCVAM 2018) as a permanent committee of the NIEHS under the National Toxicology Program Interagency Center for the Evaluation of Alternative Toxicological Methods (NICEATM). ICCVAM is composed of representatives from 16 federal regulatory and research agencies that require, use, generate, or disseminate toxicological and safety testing information. The importance of alternative research is beginning to shift from scientific to regulatory needs.

For animal welfare, the Council for International Organaization of Medical Science (CIOMS) published *International Guiding Principles for Biomedical Research Involving Animals* in 1985. This principle is proposed by scientific group and the regulatory bodies of animal welfare of many governments was accepted its concepts. These principles were revised in 2012 in conjunction with the International Council for Laboratory Animal Science (CIMOS and ICLAS 2018).

The International Standardisation Organization (ISO) also created an international document "Animal Welfare Requirement" as ISO 10993-2 in 1996 (ISO 2018). This standard is for biological and clinical evaluation of medical devices and then it is revised regularly to expand their target.

The World Animal Health Organization (OIE) is also keen to protect animal health and has introduced animal welfare as a part of animal health. The international standard of animal health (OIE Terrestrial Animal Health Code) includes not only domestic animal welfare but also research animal welfare (OIE 2018).

Asia

In Asia, the Japanese Society for Alternatives to Animal Experiments (JSAAE) was founded in 1984 as a world-first academic society consisting of scientists for alternative research (Sugawara 1990), and today JSAAE collaborates with many international organizations in this field. JSAAE is a scientific organization that undertakes research, development, education, and surveillance activities for promoting international acceptance of the 3Rs as guiding principles for the proper use of animals in scientific testing. JSAAE has published its academic journal Alternatives to Animal Testing and Experimentation (AATEX) since 1990, making it one of the oldest academic journals in this field (AATEX 2018). The society celebrated its 30th annual meeting in 2017 (JSAAE 2018).

The 6th World Congress on Alternatives was invited to Tokyo in 2006. The congress included three satellite meetings in other Asian parts, namely Beijing, Seoul and Kyoto, making it a milestone of expansion of alternative research into Asian region. Indeed, the Korean Society for Alternatives to Animal Experiments (KSAAE) was founded that same year.

The Asian Federation of Laboratory Animal Science Associations (AFLAS) is one of other remarkable activities of alternatives research. The first congress was held in Nagasaki in 2004, with subsequent meetings every two years. In 2016 the congress was hosted in Singapore (AFLAS 2018), where subjects discussed included laboratory animal welfare and 3Rs with other subjects in laboratory animal science. The AFLAS membership is now expanded to 11.

Japan

In Japan, JSAAE has a central position to propagate 3Rs activities. The initial activities of JASSE were focused on cosmetics. However, since Japan's Animal Welfare Act took 3Rs as key words, the concept has become well recognized by biomedical research organizations. The practical activities of 3Rs are held by the Japanese Association of Laboratory Animal Science (JALAS), the Japanese Society of Laboratory Animal and Environment (JSLAE), and the Japanese Association for Experimental Animal Technologists (JAEAT) as education and training sessions. Through these efforts, the 3Rs are now expanding to be recognized by industries.

Today, the 3Rs are now accepted in Asian countries widely, culminating in the first biennial Asian Congress on Alternatives being organized in 2016 in Karatsu, Japan (Asian Congress 2018). In the future, the World Congress on Alternatives is expected to be held in Asia again as well.

References

Russell WMS, Burch RL (1959) The principles of humane experimental technique. http://altweb.jhsph.edu/pubs/books/humane_exp/het-toc

FRAME (2018) History – The FRAME story. https://frame.org.uk/researching-alternatives-to-animal-testing/history/

CAAT (2018) CAAT history. http://caat.jhsph.edu/about/history.html

EURL ECVAM (2018) Home. https://eurl-ecvam.jrc.ec.europa.eu/

ICCVAM (2018) About ICCVAM. https://ntp.niehs.nih.gov/pubhealth/evalatm/iccvam/index.html

CIOMS, ICLAS (2018) International guiding principles for biomedical research involving animals. http://iclas.org/wp-content/uploads/2013/03/CIOMS-ICLAS-Principles-Final.pdf

ISO (2018) Biological evaluation of medical devices – Part 2: animal welfare requirement. https://www.iso.org/standard/36405.html

OIE (2018) Use of animals in research and education in terrestrial animal health code. http://www.oie.int/index.php?id=169&L=0&htmfile=chapitre_aw_research_education.htm

Sugawara T (1990) For the first issue of the journal AATEX 1(1):1

AATEX (2018) AATEX (Alternatives to animal testing and experimentation). http://www.asas.or.jp/jsaae/magazine/index.html. ISSN: 1344-0411

JSAAE (2018) The 30th annual meeting of the japanese society for alternatives to animal experiments 2017. http://www.asas.or.jp/jsaae/eng/events/taikai.html

AFLAS (2018) Asian federation of laboratory animal science associations. http://www.aflas-office.org/aboutus.html

Asian Congress (2018) Asian Congress 2016 on alternatives and animal use in the life science. http://www.asas.or.jp/jsaae/eng/events/asiancongress2016.html

Approaches to Reducing Animal Use for Acute Toxicity Testing: Retrospective Analyses of Pesticide Data

Judy Strickland[1(✉)], Michael W. Paris[1], David Allen[1], and Warren Casey[2]

[1] ILS, P.O. Box 13501 Research Triangle Park, Charlotte, NC 27709, USA
strickl2@niehs.nih.gov

[2] National Toxicology Program Interagency Center for the Evaluation of Alternative Toxicological Methods, National Institute of Environmental Health Sciences, P.O. Box 12233 Research Triangle Park, Charlotte, NC 27709, USA
warren.casey@nih.gov

Abstract. In this study, we considered whether acute oral toxicity hazard classifications for pesticide formulations and active ingredients (AIs) could be used to assign acute dermal toxicity hazard classifications using U.S. Environmental Protection Agency (EPA) and the United Nations Globally Harmonized System of Classification and Labelling of Chemicals (GHS) hazard categories. This retrospective analysis used highly curated acute toxicity data for 503 formulations and 297 AIs. Hazard classifications based on rat oral LD_{50} values were compared to hazard classifications based on rat dermal LD_{50} values for the same substance. The concordance of oral and dermal hazard classification was 62% for formulations and 64% for AIs using the EPA system and 71% for formulations and 55% for AIs using the GHS. Overprediction of dermal hazard was 38% for formulations and 32% for AIs using the EPA system and 28% for formulations and 41% for AIs using the GHS. Underprediction of dermal hazard was 1% for formulations and 3% for AIs using the EPA system and 1% for formulations and 3% for AIs using the GHS. While concordance overall was modest, the very low underprediction rates show that acute oral hazard categories are sufficiently protective for acute dermal hazard classification. Use of oral hazard data to also classify dermal hazard would obviate the need to perform acute dermal toxicity tests for classification and labeling and thereby reduce the number of animals used for acute systemic toxicity testing of pesticides.

Keywords: Acute toxicity · Dermal toxicity · Oral toxicity
Hazard classification

Michael W. Paris - Retired

H. Kojima et al. (Eds.): *Alternatives to Animal Testing*, pp. 37–49, 2019.
https://doi.org/10.1007/978-981-13-2447-5_5

Introduction

Dermal exposure to chemicals can occur during routine handling of chemicals or during accidental spills. Dermal exposure can contribute considerably to the internal dose of users exposed to hazardous substances [4], and in particular is an important source of internal dose for occupational chemical exposures [1, 15, 26]. For some types of chemicals, such as pesticides, the dermal route can be the most important route of exposure [12]. Because of this, the industrial hygiene community develops specific notations for substances expected to present a toxic hazard via dermal absorption [5]. Regulatory agencies use data from acute oral and dermal toxicity tests to determine the potential systemic toxicity of chemicals and chemical products following oral ingestion and topical exposure to the skin, respectively. LD_{50} values from such tests, representing the dose expected to produce lethality in 50% of the animals tested, are used to assign substances to oral and dermal hazard categories. The hazard categories are then used to assign product packaging labels to caution workers and consumers about poisoning potential.

Figures 1 and 2 show two systems for classifying substances for acute toxicity hazard. Figure 1 summarizes the hazard classification system used by the U.S. Environmental Protection Agency (EPA). EPA requires hazard labeling to be applied to pesticides with dermal or oral LD_{50} values less than or equal to 5000 mg/kg [8].

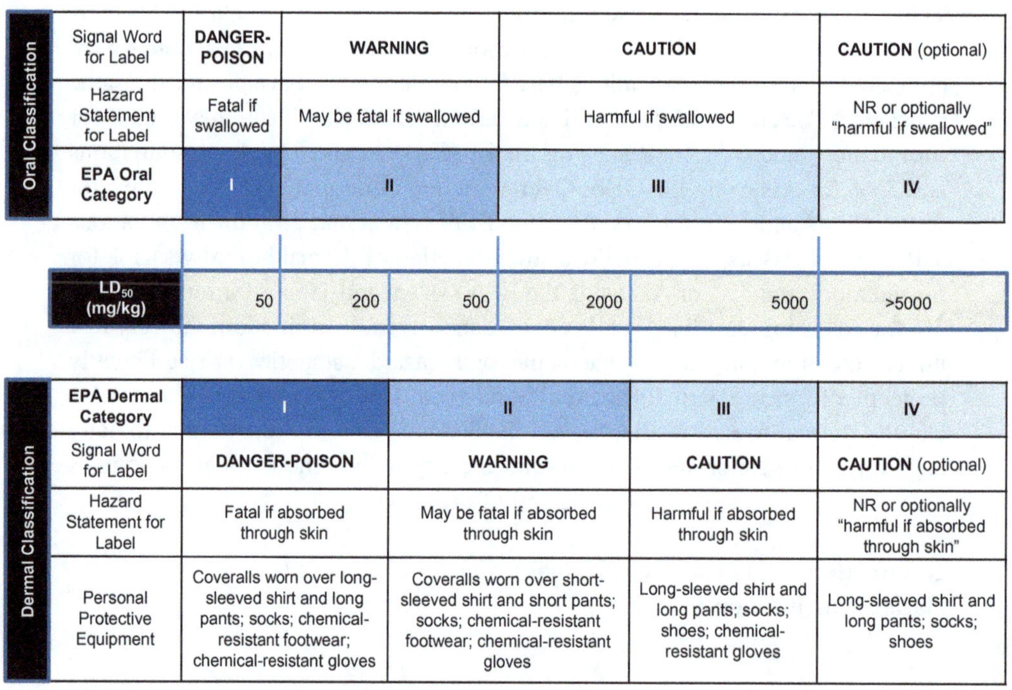

Fig. 1. EPA classification system for acute oral and dermal hazard according to the EPA Label Review Manual [8]. *NR* not required. LD_{50} dose range is not to scale Chart is adapted from Seidle et al. [27]

The EPA hazard classification system assigns a chemical to one of four oral and dermal hazard categories according to its relevant LD_{50} value, with each category associated with specific signal words and hazard statements that must be used in labeling that chemical. Dermal hazard categories are associated with specific recommendations for personal protective equipment to mitigate skin exposures.

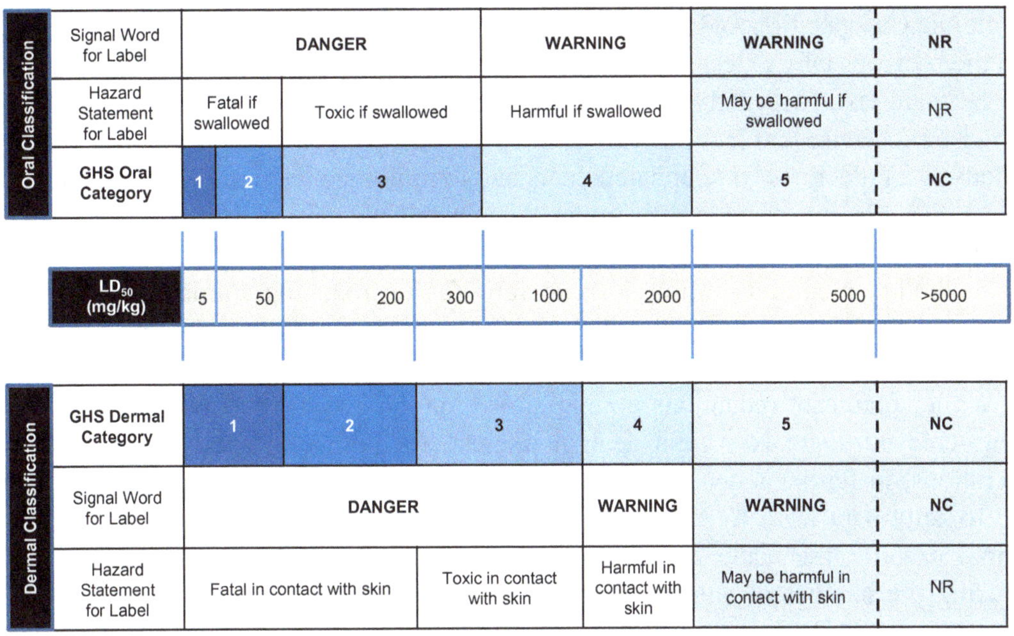

Fig. 2. GHS classifications for acute oral and dermal hazard [30]. *NR* not required, *NC* not classified. LD_{50} dose range is not to scale. The shaded category is optional and was not used for the analyses herein. Chart is adapted from Seidle et al. [27]

Figure 2 provides the requirements for labeling according to the United Nations Globally Harmonized System of Classification and Labelling of Chemicals (GHS) [30]. The GHS was established with the goal of harmonizing rules and regulations for chemical handling and labeling at the national and international levels. The GHS has five hazard categories that are associated with specific signal words and hazard statements to be used on product labels for chemicals with LD_{50} values less than or equal to 5000 mg/kg. However, Category 5, which provides for classification of chemicals having LD_{50} values greater than 2000 mg/kg but less than or equal to 5000 mg/kg, is optional. When Category 5 is not used, the GHS hazard categories provide hazard notations for chemicals with LD_{50} values less than or equal to 2000 mg/kg.

The GHS has been implemented in the European Union by Regulation No. 1272/2008 on classification, labelling and packaging of substances and mixtures, although the European Union does not use the optional Category 5 [11]. Some U.S. regulatory agencies have harmonized their classification systems with GHS. The U.S. Occupational Safety and Health Administration uses the same GHS categories as the European Union, omitting use of the optional Category 5 [25]. The U.S. Department of

Transportation uses a packing group system that is consistent with GHS Categories 1 through 3 to determine appropriate packaging and labeling of poisonous materials during transport [3].

Acute toxicity tests are the most commonly conducted product safety tests worldwide [13]. These tests can require large numbers of animals, and the animals used may experience significant pain and distress. Test methods for acute dermal systemic toxicity are described in test guidelines issued by EPA and the Organisation for Economic Co-operation and Development (OECD). The current EPA test guideline [6] and the previous OECD test guideline [17] recommend using a minimum of 20 animals for the main test. A recently revised OECD test guideline adopted in late 2017 uses a stepwise procedure that requires less than 10 animals per test [24]. Acute oral systemic toxicity test guidelines were updated years ago to minimize the number of animals used [7, 19, 20, 22] and provide refinement by minimizing pain and distress [19]. Additionally, an OECD guidance document [23] provides information on using an *in vitro* test method to predict a starting dose, thereby further reducing animal use. Currently, acute oral tests can typically use five to nine animals for main tests and five to six animals for limit tests [18].

While significant reductions in animal use for acute systemic toxicity testing have been achieved, there is a great deal of interest, for both efficiency and ethical considerations, in further reducing the number of animals used for this purpose. If acute oral toxicity data were found to be sufficient to classify pesticides for both oral and dermal hazards, the acute dermal toxicity test would then be unnecessary, thereby reducing the number of animals used for acute systemic toxicity testing. This paper describes an evaluation to determine whether acute oral toxicity classifications for pesticide formulations and active ingredients (AIs) can be used in lieu of acute dermal toxicity data for dermal hazard classification and labeling.

Materials and Methods

We collected acute oral and dermal LD_{50} data for 503 pesticide formulations and 297 AIs. To eliminate the uncertainty associated with comparing results across species, we only used LD_{50} data from acute oral and dermal tests that used rats. We obtained these data from the following sources:

- EPA Data Evaluation Reports
- EPA Reregistration Eligibility Decision documents
- Study reports submitted to fulfill EPA regulatory requirements (provided by EPA)
- Two peer-reviewed publications on acute toxicity testing of chemicals [2, 16]
- Two publicly available online toxicity databases:

    a. Hazardous Substances Data Bank [31]
    b. European Chemicals Agency database [10]

Data Quality Evaluation

Data were evaluated for reliability using Klimisch categories [14]. Only LD_{50} data with a reliability score of 1 (reliable without restriction) or 2 (reliable with restrictions) were used for our analyses. The exception was data from Creton et al. [2]; this reference indicated that the data included were reliable, but did not specify the methods used to determine reliability.

Categorization of Data

We assigned oral and dermal hazard classifications to the 503 pesticide formulations and 297 AIs according to the EPA and GHS classification systems using the respective oral and dermal LD_{50} values. We adopted the implementation of GHS that does not use the optional Category 5. Thus, substances with LD_{50} values greater than 2000 mg/kg were unclassified. If more than one LD_{50} value was available for a substance (for example, if LD_{50} values were reported for male rats, female rats, and both sexes combined), we used the lowest (i.e., most toxic) LD_{50} value to categorize the substance. When an LD_{50} was listed as greater than a specific value (e.g., greater than 2000 mg/kg), it was assigned a value just above the specific value (i.e., 2001 mg/kg for the preceding example) to assign the hazard category.

Analyses

We calculated concordance, underprediction, and overprediction rates for the classification of dermal hazard on the basis of the oral hazard classification. In these calculations, we excluded 27 formulations and 64 AIs from EPA classification because of the uncertainty of their dermal hazard classifications. These substances were characterized on the basis of limit tests as having oral LD_{50} values greater than 5000 mg/kg and dermal LD_{50} values either greater than 2000 mg/kg or greater than 4000 mg/kg. Although the oral hazard classifications for these substances were unequivocal, their dermal classifications could be either EPA dermal hazard Category III (LD_{50} greater than 2000 mg/kg but less than or equal to 5000 mg/kg) or Category IV (LD_{50} greater than 5000 mg/kg). Thus, an accurate comparison of oral and dermal hazard was not possible because the highest doses tested for the two routes were not the same. The resulting subsets of 476 formulations and 233 AIs were used for the EPA classification analyses. As noted previously, the GHS hazard classifications were determined with four hazard categories and a "not classified" category (i.e., LD_{50} greater than 2000 mg/kg). No substances were excluded from the GHS classification analyses because a substance with a dermal LD_{50} greater than 2000 mg/kg is not classified, even if the LD_{50} is actually greater than 5000 mg/kg. Thus, the full data sets of 503 formulations and 297 AIs were used for the GHS analyses.

Results

Distribution of Substances Among Hazard Categories

Figure 3 shows that, according to both the EPA and GHS hazard classifications, formulations and AIs in this data set were much more likely to be toxic via the oral route than via the dermal route, and formulations were less toxic than AIs.

EPA Hazard Categories

The majority of the formulations in our data set (70% [331/476]) were classified by the EPA system as Category IV for dermal hazard (dermal LD_{50} greater than 5000 mg/kg). However, only 36% (173/476) of these substances were classified by the EPA system as Category IV for oral hazard (Fig. 3a). Similarly, 23% (54/233) of the AIs were classified by the EPA system as Category IV for dermal hazard, but only 12% (29/233) of these substances were classified as Category IV for oral hazard (Fig. 3b).

The higher toxicity of the AIs is indicated by the lower proportion of AIs in the lowest toxicity categories, compared to the formulations. A higher proportion of formulations were classified by the EPA system as Category IV for oral hazard compared to the AIs (36% [173/476] vs. 12% [29/233]), and similarly, more formulations than AIs were classified as EPA Category IV for dermal hazard (70% [331/476] vs. 23% [54/233]) (compare Figs. 3a and b).

GHS Hazard Categories

Nearly all of the formulations in our data set (98% [494/503]) were not classified by the GHS for dermal hazard (dermal LD_{50} greater than 2000 mg/kg) (Fig. 3c). As for the EPA system, a lower proportion of these substances (71% [355/503]) was not classified by GHS for oral hazard. Similarly, 86% (255/297) of the AIs were not classified by GHS for dermal hazard, but only 51% (151/297) of these substances were not classified for oral hazard (Fig. 3d).

As with the EPA system, the AIs as a group were classified by GHS as more toxic than the formulations. A higher proportion of formulations were not classified for oral hazard by GHS compared to the AIs (71% vs. 51%), and similarly, more formulations than AIs were not classified by GHS for dermal hazard (98% vs. 86%) (compare Figs. 3c and d).

Concordance of Oral and Dermal Hazard Classifications

Figure 4 compares the concordance of EPA and GHS oral and dermal hazard classifications for formulations and AIs. The EPA classifications for dermal and oral hazard were concordant for 62% (293/476) of the formulations (Fig. 4a) and 64% (150/233) of

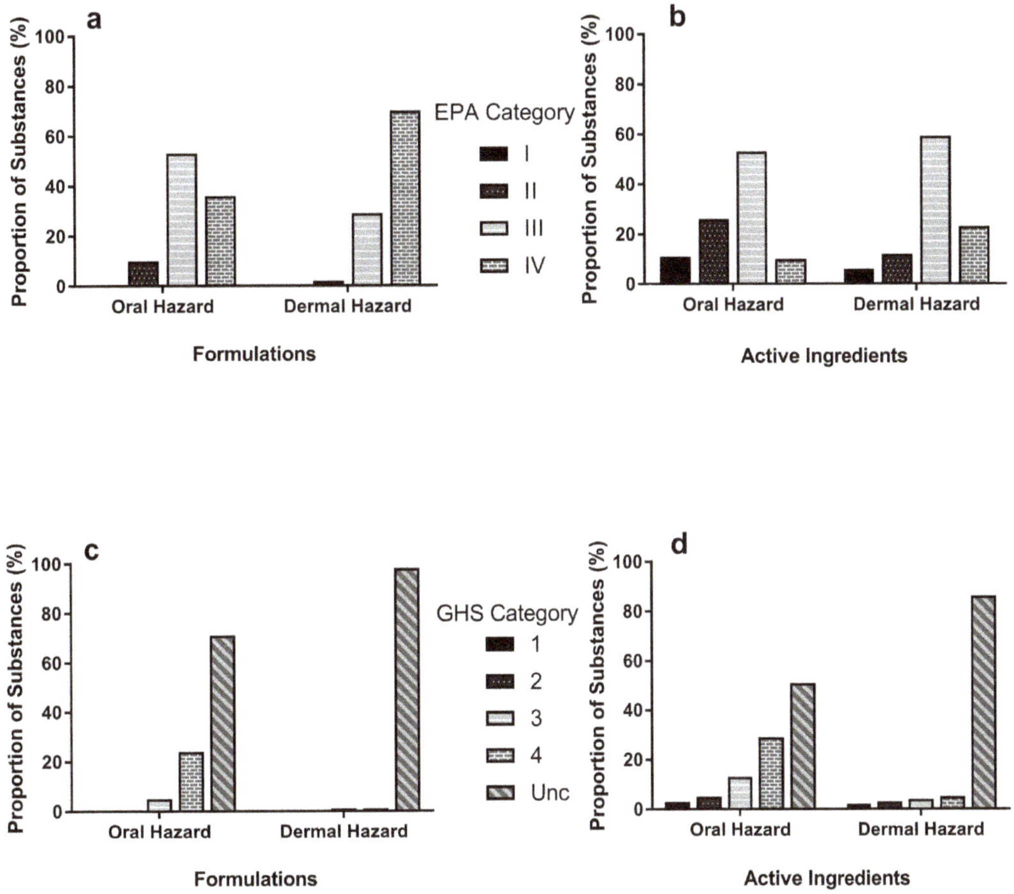

Fig. 3. Distribution of substances across EPA and GHS acute oral and dermal hazard categories. a) 476 formulations across EPA classifications b) 233 active ingredients across EPA classifications, c) 503 formulations across GHS classifications, d) 297 active ingredients across GHS classifications. *UNC* unclassified

the AIs (Fig. 4b). The EPA oral hazard classifications overpredicted dermal hazard for 38% (179/476) of the formulations and 32% (75/233) of the AIs. The EPA oral hazard classifications underpredicted dermal hazard for 1% (4/476) of the formulations and 3% (8/233) of the AIs.

The GHS classifications for dermal and oral hazard were concordant for 71% (358/503) of the formulations (Fig. 4c) and 55% (164/297) of the AIs (Fig. 4d). The GHS oral hazard classifications overpredicted dermal hazard for 28% (142/503) of the formulations and 41% (123/297) of the AIs. The GHS oral hazard classifications underpredicted dermal hazard for 1% (3/503) of the formulations and 3% (10/297) of the AIs.

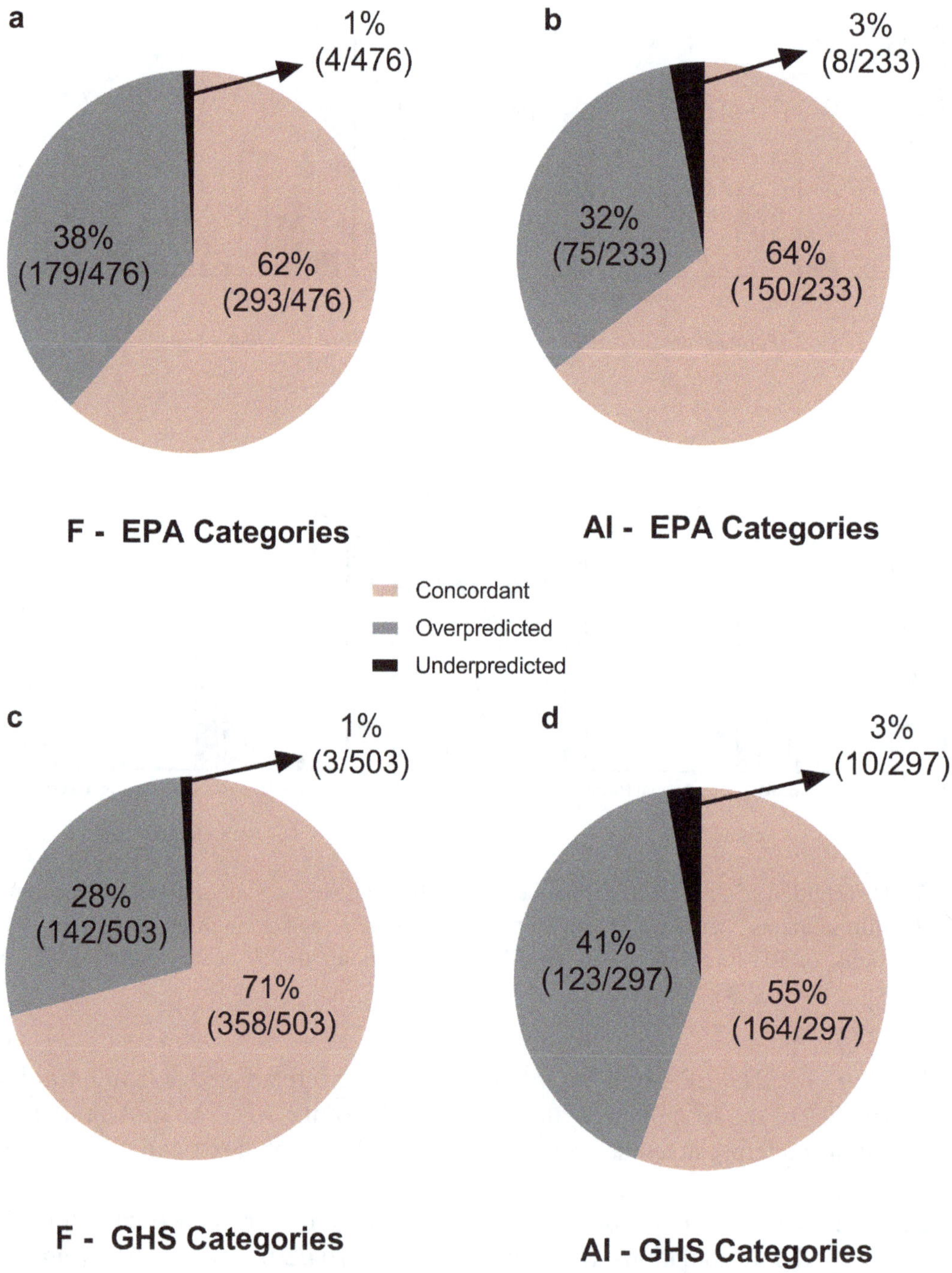

Fig. 4. Performance of oral hazard classification for predicting dermal hazard classification. Performance using the EPA classification system is shown with: a) 476 formulations and b) 233 active ingredients. Performance using the GHS classification system is shown with: c) 503 formulations and d) 297 active ingredients. *F* formulations

Discussion

Regulatory acceptance of any new alternative test method or approach requires that the new method or approach provide equivalent or better protection of human health [21, 28]. We conducted the current analysis of the use of acute oral hazard classification to classify substances for dermal hazard primarily to determine if there are instances where the acute dermal hazard is greater than the acute oral hazard. When the acute dermal toxicity hazard is greater than the acute oral toxicity hazard, the dermal hazard would be underpredicted by the oral hazard classification if that were used for dermal hazard classification. However, if such cases are rare or nonexistent, the use of oral hazard classification to predict dermal hazard would be at least as protective as using dermal LD_{50} data for this purpose because all of the predictions would either be concordant or would overpredict dermal hazard. Therefore, oral hazard categories could be used to determine dermal hazard classification without compromising public health, and product labeling could be based on the oral hazard without the need for an acute dermal systemic toxicity test.

Our analysis, which focused on the EPA hazard classification system and primarily included substances of interest to the EPA, found that using oral hazard classifications to predict dermal hazard classifications resulted in very few substances being underpredicted for dermal hazard. This is consistent with similar analyses conducted by other investigators [2, 16, 27]. Our reanalyses of these investigators' data, to the extent such data were available, provide further support for this conclusion.

Using a data set of 240 pesticide AIs, Creton et al. [2] showed that oral hazard underpredicted dermal hazard for only 0.8% (2/240) of the substances using the obsolete United Kingdom (UK) Chemicals (Hazard Information and Packaging for Supply) Regulations system [29]. The UK system was a four-category hazard classification system. Like GHS without the optional Category 5, the UK system did not classify substances with LD_{50} values greater than 2000 mg/kg as hazards, but the UK LD_{50} ranges for the other hazard categories were different from those used by the GHS. Because Creton et al. provided the dermal and oral LD_{50} data for the AIs, we were able to analyze them using the GHS and the EPA system. For our analysis of these data using the EPA system, we excluded substances with oral LD_{50} values greater than 5000 mg/kg and dermal LD_{50} values greater than 2000 mg/kg, as we did for our analysis. The underprediction rates for both EPA and GHS categories were very similar to those of our data set, which includes the Creton et al. data (Table 1).

In an analysis of a different set of 337 pesticide AIs using the same four GHS hazard categories we used, Seidle et al. [27] obtained concordance and underprediction rates similar to our AI analysis. Because this paper did not include LD_{50} data, we were not able to reanalyze their data to determine the concordance, underprediction, and overprediction rates for the classification of dermal hazard on the basis of the oral hazard classification using the EPA system.

Moore et al. [16] analyzed a broader data set of 335 substances, which included 110 pesticide AIs from Creton et al. [2] and 225 uncharacterized substances from the European Chemicals Agency database. Table 1 shows that concordance achieved by Moore et al. using GHS was much lower than ours and those of the other studies, and that their underprediction rates were higher. Our dataset consisted of only pesticide formulations and AIs. The higher underprediction and overprediction rates and lower concordance for the Moore et al. analysis could be due to inclusion of the uncharacterized substances, which comprised approximately 67% of their database. Again, because this paper did not include LD_{50} data, we were not able to reanalyze this data set to determine concordance using the EPA classification system.

While underprediction of dermal hazard would pose a clear danger to users, overprediction of dermal hazard is also undesirable, as overuse of stringent hazard warnings has a desensitizing effect, ultimately causing users to disregard them. The categorization approaches for our data sets showed that dermal hazard might be overpredicted by the oral hazard classification for 38% (179/476) of formulations using the EPA system and 28% (142/503) of formulations using the GHS (Fig. 4a, c). Similarly, rates for overprediction of dermal hazard for AIs were 32% (75/233) with the EPA system and 41% (123/297) with GHS (Fig. 4b, d).

The consequences of underprediction are more severe. Underprediction of dermal hazard could lead to warning labels and protective equipment recommendations inadequate to protect exposed persons, resulting in increased public health risk. Underprediction of dermal hazard would also affect the caution and care with which users handle consumer products. However, because dermal hazard classifications for only a small proportion of formulations (1%) and AIs (3%) in our dataset were underpredicted by using oral hazard data, our analyses suggest that acute oral hazard would provide appropriate recommendations for personal protective equipment for all but a small number of substances. If acute oral hazard were used to predict acute dermal hazard, animal testing for acute dermal toxicity would be necessary for few substances.

Our analyses, along with the others discussed here, indicate that it may be feasible to greatly reduce the use of animals for acute dermal toxicity testing of pesticide formulations and AIs. Based on the EPA acute dermal toxicity test guideline [6], waiving the dermal acute toxicity test and using oral hazard classification to assign dermal hazard classification would reduce the number of animals by 10 animals per pesticide for a limit test and 20 animals per pesticide for a main test.

EPA has used an analysis similar to ours to support guidance for waiving all acute dermal LD_{50} studies for pesticide formulations when acute oral LD_{50} studies are available [9]. Because EPA receives hundreds of acute dermal submissions for formulations each year, this development has the potential to reduce animal use significantly for acute toxicity testing. Although EPA has not waived the dermal test requirement for AIs, the waiver for formulations has a much larger impact on animal savings because the vast majority of new data submissions support registrations for formulations rather than AIs.

Future efforts to further reduce animal use for acute toxicity testing of pesticide formulations and AIs should be directed towards developing approaches to identify the small number of substances that might be underpredicted by acute oral toxicity testing before dermal tests are performed. *In silico* investigations of route-specific bioavailability could assist in identifying those substances. For substances that are likely to be

Table 1. Comparison of oral and dermal hazard concordance analyses

Oral-dermal hazard comparison	Analysis			
	Current analysis	Creton et al. [2]	Seidle et al. [27]	Moore et al. [16]
GHS concordance	55% (164/297)	40% (96/240)	54% (183/337)	17% (56/335)
GHS underprediction rate	3% (10/297)	4% (10/240)	2% (6/337)	7% (24/335)
EPA concordance	64% (150/233)	64% (116/182)	NA	NA
EPA underprediction rate	3% (8/233)	4% (7/182)	NA	NA

NA data not available "Current analysis" refers to the analysis described in this paper. Concordance and underprediction rates for Creton et al. were calculated by us from data provided in their paper. Concordance and underprediction rates for the other papers were as reported; we were not able to calculate EPA concordance and underprediction rates for these data sets because LD_{50} data were not provided in the papers

more toxic dermally than orally and must be tested using the acute dermal toxicity test, the OECD test guideline has recently been revised to use a stepwise procedure that requires fewer than 10 animals [24].

Disclaimer

This article may be the work product of an employee or group of employees of NIEHS, NIH, or other organizations. However, the statements, opinions or conclusions contained therein do not necessarily represent the statements, opinions, or conclusions of NIEHS, NIH, U.S. government, or other organizations. ILS staff do not represent NIEHS, the National Toxicology Program, or the official positions of any federal agency.

Acknowledgements. This project was funded in part with federal funds from the National Institute of Environmental Health Sciences (NIEHS), National Institutes of Health (NIH) under Contract No. HHSN273201500010C to ILS in support of the National Toxicology Program Interagency Center for the Evaluation of Alternative Toxicological Methods. The authors thank Catherine Sprankle, ILS, for editing the manuscript.

References

1. Boeniger MF, Lushniak BD (2000) Exposure and absorption of hazardous materials through the skin. Int J Occup Environ Med 6(2):148–150
2. Creton S, Dewhurst IC, Earl LK et al (2010) Acute toxicity testing of chemicals—Opportunities to avoid redundant testing and use alternative approaches. Crit Rev Toxicol 40 (1):50–83

3. DOT (2011) Hazardous Materials Regulations, 49 CFR 173
4. Drexler H (1998) Assignment of skin notation for MAK values and its legal consequences in Germany. Int Arch Occup Environ Health 71(7):503–505
5. Drexler H (2003) Skin protection and percutaneous absorption of chemical hazards. Int Arch Occup Environ Health 76:359–361
6. EPA (1998) Health effects test guidelines: OPPTS 870.1200 - Acute Dermal Toxicity, EPA 712-C-98-192. U.S. Environmental Protection Agency, Washington, DC
7. EPA (2002) Health effects test guidelines: OPPTS 870.1100 - Acute Oral Toxicity, EPA 712-C-03-197. U.S. Environmental Protection Agency, Washington, DC
8. EPA (2016a) Label review manual, office of pesticide programs. U.S. Environmental Protection Agency, Washington, DC
9. EPA (2016b) Guidance for waiving acute dermal toxicity tests for pesticide formulations & supporting retrospective analysis, office of pesticide programs. U.S. Environmental Protection Agency, Washington, DC
10. European Chemicals Agency (2017) Registered substances. https://echa.europa.eu/information-on-chemicals/registered-substances Accessed 12 Dec 2017
11. European Union (2008) Regulation (EC) No. 1272/2008 of the European Parliament and of the Council of 16 December 2008 on classification, labelling and packaging of substances and mixtures, amending and repealing Directives 67/548/EEC and 1999/45/EC, and amending Regulation (EC) No. 1907/2006, Official Journal of the European Union, L353:1-1355
12. Grandjean P (1990) Skin penetration: hazardous chemicals at work. Taylor & Francis, London
13. ICCVAM (2008) The NICEATM-ICCVAM Five-Year Plan (2008–2012): a plan to advance alternative test methods of high scientific quality to protect and advance the health of people, animals and the environment, NIH Publication No. 08-6410, National Institute of Environmental Health Sciences, Research Triangle Park, NC
14. Klimisch HJ, Andreae M, Tillmann U (1997) A systematic approach for evaluating the quality of experimental toxicological and ecotoxicological data. Regul Toxicol Pharmacol 25 (1):1–5
15. Lavoue J, Milon A, Droz PO (2008) Comparison of indices proposed as criteria for assigning skin notation. Ann Occup Hyg 52(8):747–756
16. Moore NP, Andrew DJ, Bjerke DL et al (2013) Can acute dermal systemic toxicity tests be replaced with oral tests? A comparison of route-specific systemic toxicity and hazard classifications under the globally harmonized system of classification and labelling or chemicals (GHS). Regul Toxicol Pharmacol 66:30–37
17. OECD (1987) Test no. 402: acute dermal toxicity, in OECD guidelines for the testing of chemicals, Section 4. Health Effects, Organisation for Economic Co-operation and Development, Paris
18. OECD (2001) OECD series on testing and assessment number 24, Guidance document on acute oral toxicity testing, ENV/JM/MONO(2001)4. Organisation for Economic Co-operation and Development, Paris
19. OECD (2002a) Test no. 420: acute oral toxicity - fixed dose procedure, in OECD guidelines for the testing of chemicals, Section 4. Health Effects, Organisation for Economic Co-operation and Development, Paris
20. OECD (2002b) Test no. 423: acute oral toxicity - acute toxic class method, in OECD guidelines for the testing of chemicals, Section 4. Health Effects, Organisation for Economic Co-operation and Development, Paris

21. OECD (2005) OECD series on testing and assessment number 34. Guidance document on the validation and international acceptance of new or updated test methods for hazard assessment, ENV/JM/MONO(2005)14. Organisation for Economic Co-operation and Development, Paris
22. OECD (2008) Test no. 425: acute oral toxicity: up-and-down-procedure, in OECD guidelines for the testing of chemicals, Section 4. Health Effects, Organisation for Economic Co-operation and Development, Paris
23. OECD (2010) OECD series on testing and assessment no. 129. Guidance document on using cytotoxicity tests to estimate starting doses for acute oral systemic toxicity tests, ENV/JM/MONO(2010)20. Organisation for Economic Co-operation and Development, Paris
24. OECD (2017) Test no. 402: acute dermal toxicity, in OECD guidelines for the testing of chemicals, Section 4. Health Effects, Organisation for Economic Co-operation and Development, Paris
25. OSHA (Occupational Safety and Health Administration) (2012) Occupational safety and health standards, toxic and hazardous substances. Health Hazard Criteria, 29 CFR 1910.1200 Appendix A
26. Sartorelli P, Ahlers HW, Cherrie JW et al (2010) The 2008 ICOH workshop on skin notation. La Medicina del Lavoro 101(1):3–8
27. Seidle T, Prieto P, Bulgheroni A (2011) Examining the regulatory value of multi-route mammalian acute systemic toxicity studies. Altex 28(2):95–101
28. Stokes WS, Schechtman LM (2008) Validation and regulatory acceptance of new, revised, and alternative toxicological methods. In: Hayes AW (ed) Principles and methods of toxicology, 5th edn. CRC Press, Boca Raton, pp 1103–1130
29. UK (2002) The chemicals (hazard information and packaging for supply) regulations 2002. http://www.legislation.gov.uk/uksi/2002/1689/contents/made. Accessed 11 July 2017
30. United Nations (2015) Globally harmonized system of classification and labelling of chemicals, 6th revised edn. United Nations, New York
31. U.S. National Library of Medicine (2017) Hazardous substances data bank (HSDB). https://toxnet.nlm.nih.gov/cgi-bin/sis/htmlgen?HSDB. Accessed 10 July 2017

Progress in Eliminating One-Year Dog Studies for the Safety Assessment of Pesticides

Horst Spielmann(✉)

Faculty of Biology, Chemistry and Pharmacy, Institute of Pharmacy, Freie Universität Berlin, Königin Luise Str. 2-4, 14195 Berlin, Germany
horst.spielmann@fu-berlin.de

Abstract. We reviewed six key peer-reviewed publications that assessed the need for one-year studies of pesticide toxicity in dogs. Each of the six papers took a different approach to comparing the value of one-year studies relative to three-month studies, and despite the adoption of different databases and approaches, each study reached the same conclusion: the recommended limit to the testing of pesticide toxicity in dogs should be three months.

Therefore, the present review supports the conclusion that the routine inclusion of a one-year dog study should not be a mandatory requirement for the safety assessment of pesticides, since it is scientifically no longer justifiable. We recommend that the OECD should adapt a harmonized approach that is in line with the legislation in Europe and the USA.

Keywords: Safety testing of pesticides · Regulatory testing · Dog studies Length of studies · NOAEL

Introduction and Objective

Assessment of user safety and consumer safety is a key element in the development of crop protection products and their active ingredients. Conventionally, toxicity tests using laboratory animals have been the standard means for assessing potentially hazardous effects of the chemicals used in drugs, pesticides, and consumer products like food and feed. Testing in animals has long been criticized, and the publication in 1959 of Russell and Burch's Three Rs (Russell and Burch 1959) laid the groundwork that eventually led to the banning of animal tests for the safety assessment of cosmetics in the EU (EU Commission 2009a). Moreover, since safety testing using monkeys and companion animals, such as cats and dogs, has always been the target of criticism, scientists tend to avoid using these species in testing for regulatory purposes. Consequently, although safety studies using dogs are still conducted for pesticides and drugs, they are no longer mandatory for other consumer products. Therefore, my colleagues and I at the German Federal Institute for Risk Assessment (BfR) have tried to assess

Presented at the First Asian Congress on Alternatives and Animal Use in the Life Sciences Karatsu Civic Hall in Karatsu, Saga, Fukuoka, Japan on 16 Nov 2016.

H. Kojima et al. (Eds.): *Alternatives to Animal Testing*, pp. 50–56, 2019.
https://doi.org/10.1007/978-981-13-2447-5_6

whether or not dog studies are a truly necessary means for the safety assessment of pesticides, and if they are, which types of dog studies should be used.

For the registration of pesticides repeat-dose studies with rodents and dogs have been essential elements for more than 50 years. According to international (OECD, EU) and national (US EPA and many others) test guidelines 90-day and one-year oral studies in rodents and dogs are the established standards for evaluating toxicity of pesticides. Testing typically consists of initial exploratory studies across a range of different concentrations to establish a dose that is then used in the three-month and one-year toxicity studies. Since at least 70 dogs are used to test each new chemical, and dozens of new chemicals are tested each year, the total number of animals needed quickly reaches the thousands. In recent years, changes to regulatory requirements have eliminated the need for one-year dog studies in the EU (EU Commission 2009b), and they are now required in the US, Canada, (Health Canada PMRA 2016; Linke et al. 2017) and Australia only when it can be demonstrated that dogs are more sensitive than rodents in 90-day studies.

Nevertheless, South Korea, Japan, and other countries still require a one-year dog study before a product can be approved, and this means that companies must conduct the study to be able to market the product in those countries, irrespective of the fact such testing is not required elsewhere.

The purpose of this review is to critically evaluate the need for three-months and one-year dog studies of toxicity and in particular to determine the importance, which of each of these dog studies has for the safety assessment of pesticides.

Review of Regulatory Data not in the Public Domain

For more than 50 years a three-months and a one-year dog study have been mandatory for the global registration of pesticides. It is the purpose of the studies is to identify the dose at which no adverse effects occur, this is the “no observed adverse effect level” (NOAEL), which is then used for setting a safe reference dose for humans in order to enable a risk assessment.

The toxicity data used in safety studies is obtained from testing performed by private enterprise and submitted to regulatory agencies in confidential reports. In other words, they are not in the public domain and cannot be readily obtained for other scientific purposes, such as evaluating the extent to which dog studies are actually necessary for determining a NOAEL. And in spite of the fact that such evaluations important for scientific, animal welfare, and economic purposes, proprietary toxicity data cannot be obtained or used for such purposes without the consent of the owners of the reports, e.g., agrochemical companies.

As a regulatory scientist at the Federal Institute for Risk Assessment (BfR) in Germany, which is also the national agency for the regulation of pesticides, I was able to request permission from the owners of such data and from my colleagues in the pesticides administration of the BfR to conduct an evaluation of the extent to which dog studies are necessary to the safety assessment of pesticides. In order to protect the confidentiality of the data, the chemicals had to be coded for use in the study. Although the same data is held in the files of regulatory agencies in all EU member states, Japan, and the US EPA, proprietary data on pesticides had never before been used for this type of study. In fact, the only agency that later followed our example and conducted a similar study was the US EPA. Consequently, there are only the three studies from our group at the BfR in Germany (Gerbracht and Spielmann 1998; Box and Spielmann 2005; Spielmann and Gerbracht 2001) and the three studies from the USA, in which the EPA was engaged (Baetcke et al. 2005; Doe et al. 2006; US 2006). Together with the 232 pesticides we analyzed in the German studies, the US EPA studies included both these same 232 chemicals and roughly 150 additional ones, which suggests that dog studies have been conducted for approximately no more than 380 chemicals. Unfortunately, not all the reports submitted for regulatory purposes included data from rodent studies, which would be a prerequisite in order to determine the NOAEL for pesticides using long-term rodent studies alone or by combining long-term rodent studies with short-term dog studies, rather than just long-term dog studies.

Results of the Studies Conducted in Germany

The results of the safety reports submitted to the BfR in Germany for 232 pesticides (Gerbracht and Spielmann 1998; Spielmann and Gerbracht 2001; Box and Spielmann 2005) provided two major conclusions:

1. The testing of pesticides in dogs is indeed necessary because the dog has proved to be the most sensitive species for about 15% of the compounds examined.
2. Chronic studies are of limited value, since they provide essential information that cannot be obtained in sub-chronic studies only in about 5% of all cases.

These conclusions are corroborated by several retrospective analyses of safety studies on pharmaceutical drugs carried out in the context of the International Conference on Harmonization (ICH) for the registration of pharmaceuticals for human use. Over 90% of the drugs test elicited no toxic symptoms in one-year dog studies that were conducted in addition to prior 90- or 180-day dog or rodent studies. Another approach, in which the results from pre-clinical animal studies were compared with those from clinical studies, demonstrated that animal studies predicted about 70% of the effects observed in volunteers, and that in about 94% of the cases, these effects occurred in animal studies lasting no more than one month.

Based on these results, the report recommended abandoning the regulatory requirement for the routine carrying out of one-year dog studies. Also, while 90-day studies should be conducted in both dogs and rodents, chronic studies should only take place in rodents. In cases where dogs are more sensitive than rodents in the 90-day study, rather than conducting a one-year dog study, an additional safety factor should be applied to the NOAEL value obtained in the chronic rodent study in order to set an appropriate threshold for safe human exposure. This safety factor may be calculated from chronic NOAEL data available from several pesticide databases. Chronic tests using dogs would then only be required if the test compound belongs to a new class of chemicals that has never been tested before. Thus, the report concludes that, according to current scientific knowledge, routine one-year dog studies are no longer required for agricultural chemicals and pesticides, and international regulations should be changed accordingly. Active international support of such measures is welcomed from both an economic and an animal-welfare perspective.

Results of the Studies Conducted by the US EPA

The review performed by Baetcke et al. (2005) was based on a comprehensive database of registered compounds that is maintained by the US EPA. The authors showed for 77 compounds that data from dog studies had an impact on the derivation of reference doses.

The authors of the study concluded: *"Thus the present analysis indicates that a 13-week dog study would be adequate for identification of a NOAEL or LOAEL that would be similar to that established from a chronic dog study except 3 pesticides (3/77or 4%) of the cases evaluated."* And *"Thus, the results of this current retrospective analysis of studies on pesticides, when considered with the results of the analysis by* Spielmann and Gerbracht (2001), *show, with few exceptions, that a 13-week dog study is as adequate as a 1-year dog study for identification of a NOAEL."*

In 2006 the US EPA conducted additional analyses of dog studies conducted with pesticide chemicals (*Length of Dog Toxicity Study(ies) that is Appropriate for Chronic RfD Determinations of Pesticide Chemicals)*. In this analysis a total of 110 pesticides representing more than 50 classes were scrutinized.

The authors of the study concluded: *"This larger analysis supports the conclusion that longer-duration studies (one year) in the dog do not result in appreciably lower NOAELs or identify new effects for the majority of chemicals when compared to the shorter-duration study 13-week study in this species. Thus, reliance on the required chronic rodent studies, two-generation rat reproductive study, and the thirteen-week dog toxicity study is generally expected to provide an adequate basis for chronic NOEL derivation in pesticide risk assessment. EPA acknowledges that there may be situations where a longer duration dog toxicity study may be warranted when a pesticide chemical is highly bio-accumulating (e.g. builds up in body fat) and is eliminated so slowly that it does not achieve steady state or sufficient tissue concentrations to elicit an effect during a 90-day study. EPA anticipates that this situation will be infrequent since current pesticides are not usually designed to be highly persistent and bio-accumulating. If such a chemical is encountered, EPA would require the appropriate tier 2 metabolism and pharmacokinetic studies to more precisely evaluate bioavailability, half-life, and steady state and determine if a longer duration dog toxicity study is needed."*

Based on this conclusion, the US EPA removed the one-year study in dogs from the list of studies required for the regulation of pesticides.

Relevance of the One-Year Dog Study in Assessing Human Health Risks for Registration of Pesticides. An Update to Include Pesticides Registered in Japan

A recent publication by Kobel et al. (2014) focused on Japan, which is considered a key region, and demonstrated the redundancy of the one-year dog study for agrochemical testing based on an analysis of data on the 400+ pesticides registered in that region. The setting of a so-called Acceptable Daily Intake (ADI), which defines limits on the amount of any particular chemical that a human should be exposed to over a lifetime, is a key means of protecting human health. ADIs derived from dog studies are available for 45 of these 400 pesticides, and these 45 ADIs were analyzed in detail. The study showed that excluding data from the one-year dog studies would have made no real difference in the setting of exposure limits for over 90% of these 45 pesticides. Additionally, there might have been a difference in 6.5% of the cases, and there would have been a genuine difference in the ADI recommendation in only 2.2% of the cases, which is to say, one chemical.

The retrospective data analysis showed that, in 99% of cases there would have been no significant impact on the safe exposure levels derived in Japan had the one-year dog studies not been conducted, and that in all cases consumer exposure would have remained well below the ADI.

This key publication adds substantially to the weight of published literature now indicating that one-year dog studies add no significant value to the safety assessment of agrochemicals. European regulations no longer require one-year dog studies. We now need to work towards a harmonized approach with countries in other parts of the world. The time has come for one-year dog studies to be removed from test requirements globally.

Discussion

The limitations of each of these reviews are well understood as is the need for greater comprehensiveness, and Baetcke et al. (2005) have asked for a broader review of entire databases, not just the chemicals for which dog studies drive the safety assessment. In response to this, the US EPA performed an extensive review in 2006 and concluded that for pesticide risk assessment dog studies should be conducted for more than three months. There is no disputing the need for repeat-dose studies in dogs of three months' duration. The weight of evidence, however, of all these reviews together—and in particular the studies conducted in dogs (Gerbracht and Spielmann 1998; Spielmann and Gerbracht 2001; Box and Spielmann 2005; Doe et al. 2006; Baetcke et al. 2005; Kobel et al. 2010; US 2006)—shows conclusively that there is little value in conducting a one-year dog study in addition to a three-month study, which strongly suggests that such studies can be safely eliminated from the list of studies that are mandatory for the safety assessment of pesticides. Of all the chemicals in the databases analyzed in the four main publications critically reviewed here, only 3–4% had reference doses the setting of which was influenced by the results of a one-year dog study.

We consider the combined weight of evidence from these four reviews clearly demonstrates that dog studies for pesticides need be no more than three months long. The fact that each review arrived at a similar conclusion despite having taken a different approach to the subject matter provides additional support for our conclusion. In cases where dogs are apparently more sensitive than rodents in three-month studies a comparative evaluation for kinetics, and differences in dynamics should be analyzed.

Evidence from all of these reviews as well as from their combined consideration supports the conclusion that dog studies are necessary but can be limited to three months' duration without compromising human safety. Thus, as suggested in some of the reviews, improvements in study design are called for. Therefore, a balanced consideration from the scientific and animal welfare perspectives suggests that national requirements which are insisting on one-year dog studies for the regulation of pesticides should be updated in order to be in line with the regulations established in the EU and the USA, which would eliminate the requirements for dog studies longer than 3 months' duration.

References

Baetcke KP, Phang W, Dellarco V (2005) A comparison of the results of studies on pesticides from 12- or 24-month dog studies with shorter duration. US EPA, 4/7/05. http://www.epa.gov/scipoly/sap/meetings/2005/may2/dogstudymay05.pdf

Box RJ, Spielmann H (2005) Use of dog the dog as non-rodent species in the safety testing schedule associated with the registration of crop and plant protection products (pesticides): present status. Arch Toxicol 79:615–626

Doe JE, Boobis AR, Blaker A, Dellarco V, Doerrer NG, Franklin C, Goddman JI, Kronenberg JM, Lewis R, McConnel EE, Mercier T, Moretto A, Nolan C, Padilla S, Phang W, Solecki R, Tilbury L, van Ravenzwaay B, Wolf DC (2006) A tiered approach to systemic toxicity testing for agricultural chemical safety assessment. Crit Rev Toxicol 36:37–68

EU Commission (2009a) Regulation (EC) No 1223/2009 of the European Parliament and of the Council of 30 November 2009 on Cosmetic Products

EU Commission (2009b) Regulation (EC) No 1107/2009 of the European Parliament and of the Council of 21 October 2009 concerning the placing of plant protection products on the market and repealing Council Directives 79/117/EEC and 91/414/EEC

Gerbracht U, Spielmann H (1998) The use of dogs as second species in regulatory testing of pesticides: I. Interspecies comparison. Arch Toxicol 72:319–329

Health Canada Pest Management Regulatory Agency (HC PMRA) (2016) Guidance for developing datasets for conventional pest control product applications: data codes for parts 1, 2, 3, 4, 5, 6, 7 and 10. http://www.hc-sc.gc.ca/cps-spc/pubs/pest/_pol-guide/data-guide-donnees/index-eng.php

Kobel W, Feger I, Billing R, Lewis R, Bentley K, Bomann W, Botham P, Stahl B, van Revenzwaay B, Spielmann H (2010) A 1-year toxicity study in dogs is no longer a scientifically justifiable core data requirement for the safety assessment of pesticides. Crit Rev Toxicol 40:1–15

Kobel W, Fegert I, Billington R, Lewis E, Bentley K, Langrand-Lerche C, Botham P, Sato M, Debruyne E, Strupp C, van Ravenzwaay B (2014) Relevance of the 1-year dog study in assessing human health risks for registration of pesticides. An update to include pesticides registered in Japan. Crit Rev Toxicol 44:842–848

Linke B, Mohr S, Ramsingh D, Bhuller Y (2017) A retrospective analysis of the added value of 1-year dog studies in pesticide human health risk assessments. Crit Rev Toxicol 47:587–597

Russell WMS, Burch RL (1959) The principles of humane experimental technique. Methuen & Co. Ltd., London

Spielmann H, Gerbracht U (2001) The use of dogs as second species in regulatory testing of pesticides. Part II. Subacute, subchronic and chronic studies in the dog. Arch Toxicol 75:1–21

US EPA (2006) Length of Dog Toxicity Study(ies) that is Appropriate for Chronic RfD Determinations of Pesticide Chemicals. Washington, DC: Health Effects Division, Office of Pesticide Programs, US Environmental Protection Agency. March 20, 2006

Cosmetic Regulation and Alternatives to Animal Experimentation in India

Mohammad A. Akbarsha[1,2(✉)] and Benedict Mascarenhas[3]

[1] Life Sciences Research, National College (Autonomous), Tiruchirappalli 620001, India
akbarbdu@gmail.com
[2] Mahatma Gandhi – Doerenkamp Center for Alternatives, Bharathidasan University, Tiruchirappalli 620 024, India
[3] EnvisBE Solutions Pvt. Ltd, Dadar (West), Mumbai 400028, India
ben_mas@envisbesolutions.com

Abstract. United Kingdom was the first to ban animal testing of cosmetics, and it happened in 1998. The European Union (EU) went through legislations and endeavors implementing animal testing ban in a phased manner, and the final step was done in 2013. Consequent to this, there was enormous canvassing for ban of cosmetic testing on animals in India, to harmonize the marketing as well as import ban of EU. The Indian Drug and Cosmetic Regulatory Authority conceded the demand resulting in the final ban in 2014. This review traces the evolution of thought sequence resulting in the ban, and approval of adopting OECD Guidelines for *in vitro* testing of skin and eye irritation and corrosion.

Keywords: India · European Union · Cosmetic testing · Draize tests OECD

Introduction

The EU defines a cosmetic product as “any substance or preparation intended to be placed in contact with the various external parts of the human body (epidermis, hair system, nails, lips and external genital organs) or with the teeth and the mucous membranes of the oral cavity with a view exclusively or mainly to cleaning them, perfuming them, changing their appearance and/or correcting body odors and/or protecting them or keeping them in good condition”[1].

Cosmetics and ingredients therein, however much applied only externally, are all chemicals, some of which are known or speculated to produce adverse reactions locally and occasionally systemically in view of dermal absorption or inhalation. Therefore, the regulatory authorities of cosmetics in many countries have mandated testing of the cosmetics/ingredients for risks/adverse effects. For much of the last century this testing has been done in animals, and different animals are used in different tests; for e.g. skin and eye irritation/corrosion are tested in rabbits (Draize tests); dermal penetration, 90 day repeated oral dose, carcinogenicity, reproductive toxicity, and acute oral toxicity in

[1] www.cosmeticsinfo.org/Regulation-in-eu.

H. Kojima et al. (Eds.): *Alternatives to Animal Testing*, pp. 57–62, 2019.
https://doi.org/10.1007/978-981-13-2447-5_7

rat; skin sensitization and phototoxicity in guinea pig; genotoxicity in mouse; and phototoxicity and carcinogenicity in mouse also. In view of lack of relevance of data generated in animal models to humans in many instances, and the harm done to the animal subjects, this testing has been opposed. The awareness thus created resulted in European Union (EU) ban of cosmetic animal testing and sales in a phased manner, with the final stage falling through in 2013 [1–3]. Thereupon, towards harmonization of EU Cosmetic Regulation, several other countries- Israel, Norway, India, New Zealand, Taiwan, South Korea, Turkey, Switzerland, and Guatemala, and six states in Brazil, have banned or restricted animal testing of cosmetics [3, 4]. Similar legal measures have been proposed and are under political debate in several other countries, including the United States, Canada, Australia, and South Africa [5]. This article reviews the evolution of thought sequence in India.

History of Ban of Animal Testing of Cosmetics in EU

The EU, consisting of 28 member states, became the world's first set of countries to ban cosmetic animal testing and trade. In 1993 the 6th Amendment to EU Directive 76/768/EEC was passed and contained a ban on the sale of newly animal-tested cosmetic products. To make sure that adequate time was given to find non-animal methods, the deadline for the ban to come into effect was 1st January 1998. In 1997 the ban was delayed until 30th June 2000, and then further delayed until 30th June 2002 due to a lack of adequate validated alternative methods. In 2003 the 7th Amendment to EU Directive 76/768/EEC was passed and contained a phased-in ban on animal testing for cosmetics with a deadline of 2013: Ban on animal testing of finished products, ban on animal testing of cosmetic ingredients, ban on marketing of finished products tested on animals post-enactment, and ban on marketing of cosmetics containing ingredients tested on animals post-ban. Thus, on 11th September 2004 the ban on animal testing of finished cosmetic products came into force. The sale of cosmetic ingredients tested on animals outside the EU using methods that have been replaced within the EU was also banned. On 11th March 2009 the ban on animal testing of cosmetic ingredients within the EU was implemented. The sale of cosmetic products containing newly animal-tested ingredients was banned; however, animal testing was still allowed for complex human health issues such as repeat dose toxicity, reproductive toxicity and toxico kinetics. On 11th March 2013 the full ban came into effect and it is now illegal to market or sell cosmetics in the EU where the finished product or ingredients have been tested on animals after enactment of the relevant phase of the ban. As of 11th July 2013 EU Directive 76/768/EEC has been replaced by EU Regulation 1223/2009 (Cosmetics Regulation), which contains all the same provisions (Fig. 1). Thus, the entire endeavor took more than 20 years to reach the final phase, as of now, and of course great lot of financial input from governmental agencies and cosmetic industry partners, and a great lot of scientific deliberations [1, 3], this long time and money to ensure that adequate

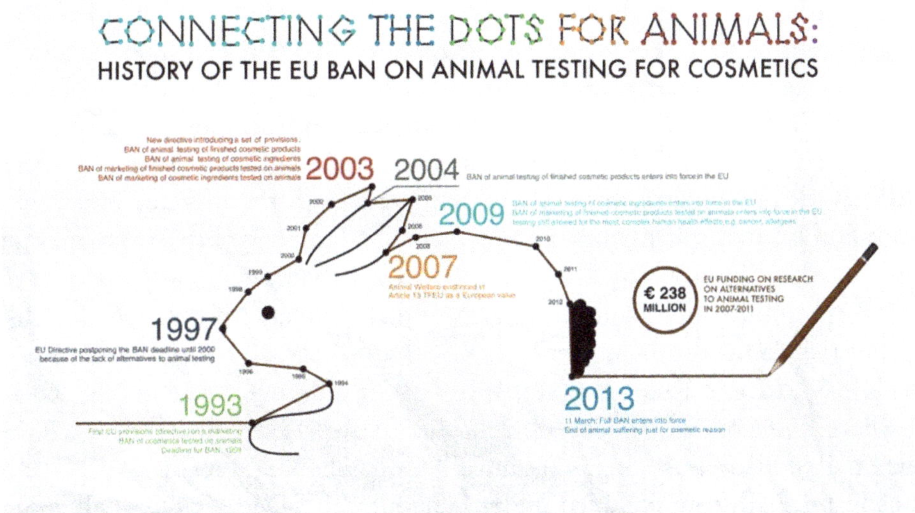

Fig. 1. Connecting the dots for animals: History of the EU ban on animal testing for cosmetics. [Adopted from www.understandinganimalresearch.org.uk/policy/cosmetics/]

and appropriate non-animal testing methods have become available. Due to the development of non-animal techniques it became apparent that these animal studies were no longer required.[2]

Cosmetic Regulation in India

The Central Drugs Standard Control Organization (CDSCO) is the Central Authority for discharging regulatory functions relating to drugs and cosmetics, assigned to the Central Government under the Drugs and Cosmetics Act, 1940 (D&C Act), and Drugs and Cosmetics Rules, 1945. It is headed by Drugs Controller General (India), headquartered in New Delhi. The vision of CDSCO is to protect and promote public health in India. It has as mission "to safeguard and enhance public health by assuring the safety, efficacy and quality of drugs, cosmetics and medical devices". Each of the 29 States and 7 Union Territories of India has its own Drug Control Authority (SDCA) headed by the Drug Controller/Commissioner/Director, who is responsible for discharging regulatory functions assigned under the provisions of the Drugs and Cosmetics Act, 1940, and Drugs and Cosmetics Rules, 1945.

The Bureau of Indian Standards (BIS) is a statutory organization under the Bureau of Indian Standards Act, 1986. The BIS formulates national standards and carries out conformity assessment by operating the Product and Management System Certification Scheme. One of the activities of BIS is to lay down standards for cosmetics in India. The Cosmetic Regulation is governed by Drugs and Cosmetics Act, 1940, and the Drugs and Cosmetics Rules, 1945, made under the Act.

---

[2] www.understandinganimalresearch.org.uk/policy/cosmetics/.

Cosmetic is defined under the D&C Act as any article intended for cleansing, beautifying, promoting attractiveness, altering the appearance and any article intended for use as a component of cosmetic. Under the said rule and law, no cosmetic can be manufactured for sale except in accordance with the conditions of manufacturing license issued by the respective SDCA. No cosmetic can be imported for sale except in accordance with the conditions of Import Registration Certificate issued by the DCGI. D&C Act and Rules require that cosmetics marketed in the country are safe and of standard quality; importort manufacture of sub-standard, misbranded, adulterated and spurious cosmetics is prohibited, and the Central Government has power under the D&C Act to prohibit manufacture or import of any cosmetic, use of which is likely to involve any risk to human beings.

Schedule-S to D&C Rules contains a list of 30 different cosmetics which include skin powders and creams, tooth powders and pastes, hair oils, powder hair dyes, shampoo, nail polish, lipstick, after-shave lotion, shaving creams, soaps, etc. The cosmetics in finished form included under Schedule-S of D&C Rules shall conform to the Indian Standards specifications laid down from time to time by the BIS. No cosmetic shall contain dyes, colours, and pigments other than those specified by the BIS (IS4707 Part 1 as amended) and Schedule-Q. The IS 4707 (Part 1) lists dyes, pigments and colors which are generally recognized as safe (GRAS) and which when used in concentrations conventionally adopted or within the limits as stipulated is permissible, and IS 4707 (Part 2) lists cosmetics raw materials and adjuncts, other than dyes, colors, and pigments in the following four groups: (A) list of substances classified as 'GRAS' which must not form part of the composition of cosmetic products -Annexure A of the standard; (B) list of substances which cosmetic products must not contain except subject to the restrictions and conditions laid down (Annexure B of the standard); (C) list of preservatives allowed (Annexure C of the standard); and (D) list of UV filters allowed in sunscreen products (Annexure D of the standard). Cosmetic products formulated as per the restrictions imposed by IS 4707 (Parts 1 and 2) and the list of Cosmetics, Toiletry and Fragrance Association (CTFA), European Economic Community (EEC) and the guidelines of Cosmetics Europe Guidelines on Exchange of Information (IFRA) are likely to be safe, and such products may not warrant any safety testing, whereas products which contain novel ingredients which are not under the purview of the above documents shall require safety testing as per the guidelines provided in IS 4011. The IS 4011: 1997 laid down by BIS prescribes "Methods of test for safety evaluation of cosmetics". Requirement of labeling of products not tested for safety on animals with the statement "The product has not been tested on animals for safety" was deleted from the Standard in 2002. Skin irritation test and eye irritation test (Draize tests in rabbits) were removed from the Standard in 2007. In February 2014, the IS 4011 was amended specifying that when there is a need for safety evaluation of cosmetic products to demonstrate absence of oral toxicity and/or oral mucosal irritation, the manufacturer shall submit the safety data based on alternative non-animal test methods to the concerned State Licensing Authorities for their consideration and approval.

Ban on Use of Animals in Cosmetic Testing

In response to public campaigning led by Humane Society International-India, PETA India, and P*f*A, the Drug Technical Advisory Board (DTAB), a statutory body under the D&C Act deliberated the issue of testing of cosmetics on animals in its 65th meeting held on 25.11.2013 and recommended prohibition of the same by amending the D&C Rules. Based on the recommendation, Government of India published a draft Rule vide G.S.R. 16(E) dated 13.01.2014 for prohibition of testing of cosmetics on animals. The draft rule was made available for public comments. After examination of the public comments, Government of India prohibited the testing of cosmetics on animals vide G.S.R. 346(E) dated 21.05.2014 by inserting the following rule in the D&C Rules, "148-C: Prohibition of testing of cosmetics on animals-No person shall use any animal for testing cosmetics". Further, it was specified that when there is a need for safety evaluation of cosmetic products to demonstrate absence of oral toxicity and/or oral mucosal irritation, the manufacturer shall submit the safety data based on alternative non-animal test methods to the concerned State Licensing Authorities for their consideration and approval [6].

Prohibition of Import of Cosmetics Tested on Animals

The Government of India published Draft Rules vide G.S.R. 311(E) dated 05.05.2014 for prohibition of import of cosmetics tested on animals. The draft rule was made available for public comments. After examination of the public comments, the Government of India amended the D&C Rules, which prohibited the import of cosmetics tested on animals vide G.S.R. 718(E) dated 13.10.2014. Further clarifications were issued on 15.02.2015 and 29.06.2015, according to which the importer should submit original undertaking from the manufacturer (legal/actual brand owner) of the registered products stating that cosmetic products have not been tested on animals on and after 12.11.2014; and new applicants should submit this undertaking along with registration dossier to CDSCO wherein copy of the undertaking may be produced at ports for clearing the consignments.

Conclusion

It is of historical importance that India has earned reputation as the first south east Asian country to implement ban of animal testing of cosmetics, finished products as well as ingredients, domestic as well as import. Yet, it may be some more time before internationally recognized non-animal testing methods are fully implemented in India, and until full non-animal replacements are available for all endpoints. As of now, the OECD non-animal guidelines for skin and eye irritation and corrosion, skin sensitization, and other endpoints are to be followed, using weight of evidence and Integrated Approaches to Testing and Assessment (IATA), in order to assess the toxicity potential of novel cosmetic ingredients or finished product.

Acknowledgments. We thank Doerenkamp-Zbinden Foundation, Switzerland, for the fund to establish Mahatma Gandhi-Doerenkamp Center for Alternatives in India, and the DCGI-Government of India, PeTA India and HSI-India, for providing some of the material in the coverage.

References

1. Adler S, Basketter D, Creton S et al (2011) Alternative (non-animal) methods for cosmetics testing: current status and future prospects-2010. Arch Toxicol 85(5):367–485
2. Hartung T, Blaauboer BJ, Bosgra S et al (2011) An expert consortium review of the EC-commissioned report alternative (non-animal) methods for cosmetics testing: current status and future prospects–2010. Altex 28(3):183–209
3. Laquieze L, Lorencini M, Granjeir JM (2015) Alternative methods to animal testing and cosmetic safety: an update on regulations and ethical considerations in Brazil. Appl In Vitro Toxicol 1(4):243–253
4. Palmer N (2015) Global cosmetic compliance summit. Global cosmetic compliance. www.globalcosmeticcompliance.com
5. Knight J, Rovida C (2014) Safety evaluations under the proposed US safe cosmetics and personal care products act of 2013: animal use and cost estimates. Altex 31(2):177–208
6. Koduri C, Akbarsha MA (2014) India: end to animal testing of cosmetics and household products. Altex 31(2):236–237

Guidance on the Use of Alternative Test Methods for the Safety Assessment of Cosmetics and Quasi-drugs

Hajime Kojima[1(✉)], Yoshiaki Ikarashi[2], Tokio Nakada[3], Akiko Yagami[4], Kenji Sugibayashi[5], Hiroaki Todo[5], Yukiko Hoshino[6], Naofumi Iizuka[6], Takatoshi Nakamura[6], Shinichi Sekizawa[6], Kazutoshi Shinoda[6], Mio Yagi[6], Daisuke Araki[7], Hitoshi Sakaguchi[7], Hitoshi Sasa[7], and Mariko Sugiyama[7]

[1] Japanese Center for the Validation of Alternative Methods (JaCVAM), National Institute of Health Sciences (NIHS), 3-25-26 Tonomachi, Kawasaki-Ku, Kawasaki, Kanagawa 210-9501, Japan
h-kojima@nihs.go.jp
[2] National Institute of Health Sciences, Kawasaki, Kanagawa, Japan
[3] Department of Dermatology, Showa University, Fujigaoka Hospital, Yokohama, Japan
[4] Department of Dermatology, Fujita Health University School of Medicine, Toyoake, Aichi, Japan
[5] Faculty of Pharmaceutical Sciences, Josai University, Sakado, Saitama, Japan
[6] Pharmaceuticals and Medical Devices Agency, Tokyo, Japan
[7] Japan Cosmetic Industry Association, Tokyo, Japan

Abstract. In accordance with a notification issued by Japan's Ministry of Health, Labour and Welfare (MHLW) in 2011, the Japanese Center for the Validation of Alternative Methods (JaCVAM) has accelerated applications for new test methods developed as alternatives to animal testing for the safety assessment of the manufacture and sales of cosmetic products and quasi-drug products that contain new ingredients. Taking advantage of this opportunity to strongly impact testing throughout Japan, researchers have been coordinating guidance on the use of such alternative test methods since 2012. Based on test guidelines issued by the Organisation for Economic Co-operation and Development (OECD) and JaCVAM evaluation documents, dermatologists and representatives of cosmetic companies as well as specialists from both the Pharmaceuticals and Medical Devices Agency (PMDA) and the National Institute of Health Sciences (NIHS) have drafted guidance documents for a number of alternative test methods.

Keywords: Cosmetic · Quasi-drug · JaCVAM · Guidance document

Presented at the First Asian Congress on Alternatives and Animal Use in the Life Sciences, Karatsu Civic Hall in Karatsu, Saga, Fukuoka, Japan on 16 Nov 2016.

H. Kojima et al. (Eds.): *Alternatives to Animal Testing*, pp. 63–68, 2019.
https://doi.org/10.1007/978-981-13-2447-5_8

A complete ban on the marketing of cosmetic products and cosmetic ingredients that have been tested on animals has been in effect in the EU since March 2013 [1]. In the light of this regulation, almost all Japanese cosmetic manufacturers have ceased the use of animal testing in the development of cosmetic products and ingredients. Just as in the EU, Japanese regulatory agencies as well as the MHLW have adopted positive and negative lists and generally do not require permits for the manufacture and sale of new cosmetic products that contain known ingredients. In cases where safety assessment of the manufacture and sales of quasi-drug products that contain new ingredients and new cosmetic ingredients is required, however, the MHLW still requires that applications for safety assessment be supported with animal data.

MHLW Updates

As shown in Table 1, the use of new cosmetic ingredients requires the submission of results from safety assessment performed with animal testing, In such cases, the test methods must ordinarily conform to notifications regarding pharmaceutical safety, OECD test guidelines, and other publicly-recognized standards. They must also appear in the *keshohin-iyakubu gaihin seizou hanbai gaidobukku 2011–2012* (the 2011–2012 Guidebook on the Manufacture and Sales of Cosmetics and Quasi-Drugs) [2]. Also, all animal testing must conform to *koseirodousho non shokan suru jisshikikan ni okeru doubutsu jiken tou no jisshi ni kan suru kihonhoushin* (Basic Policies Regarding Implementation of Animal and Other Testing at Organizations under the Jurisdiction of the MHLW), as well as all other laws and regulations relevant to animal and other testing [3].

An administrative notice [4] issued in July 2006 by the MHLW Evaluation and Licensing Division indicated that the inclusion of results from alternative test methods as documentary evidence in an application was acceptable, provided that the alternative test methods conformed to accepted OECD test methods or had been similarly validated in a suitable manner. The administrative notice further stipulated that, in cases where animal testing was to be performed, if information about the physicochemical properties of the test chemical itself or similar chemical substances as well as the results of non-animal testing (in vitro, in chemico, in silico testing) led to the reasonable expectation that the test chemicals could induce distress or suffering in test animals, efforts to mitigate such distress or suffering by diluting test chemicals would be required.

On 4 February 2011, the MHLW issued a notification that data obtained with alternative test methods approved by JaCVAM could be used for the submission of quasi-drug applications, or for petitions to include ingredients in the Standards for Cosmetics [5]. Information is available on the JaCVAM website [6] to help ensure proper preparation of the documentary evidence to be included with applications for approval of manufacturing and sales of quasi-drug products as well as in requests for revisions to the positive list for cosmetics. This information has been made available to the appropriate businesses and other concerned parties industrywide. In addition, administrative notices issued in April 2012 and May 2013 by the MHLW Evaluation and Licensing Division publicized the availability of alternative test methods for

Table 1. Test methods for regulatory use in safety assessment of ingredients in Japan

Quasi-drug safety evaluation guidance	
For main ingredients	For additives
Acute toxicity	Acute oral toxicity
Repeat dose toxicity (Sub-chronic, Chronic)	NR
Reproductive toxicity	NR
Local irritation (Skin, Mucous membrane)	Primary skin irritation
	Cumulative skin irritation
	Ocular irritation
Skin sensitization	Skin sensitization
Photo safety	Photo safety
Genotoxicity	Genotoxicity
Carcinogenicity (case by case)	NR
ADME	ADME (case by case)
Human patch test	Human patch test
Human use test	NR

NR: Not Required

phototoxicity testing and skin sensitization testing for use in safety assessment of cosmetics and quasi-drugs [5]. Additional information on other alternatives to animal testing will be issued as it becomes available. Dermatologists and representatives of cosmetic companies as well as specialists from both the PMDA and the NIHS have drafted guidance documents for a number of alternative test methods based on OECD test guidelines and JaCVAM evaluation documents.

Alternative test methods developed for OECD test guidelines are useful in predicting potential hazards of exposure to chemicals, even though they are not always suitable for providing the wide range of information needed for comprehensive safety and risk assessment. Thus, manufacturers often have difficulty gaining approval from Japanese regulators for new cosmetic ingredients unless they perform animal testing [6].

JaCVAM Update

JaCVAM was established to promote the use of alternative methods to animal testing in regulatory studies, thereby replacing, reducing, or refining the use of animals wherever possible, while meeting the responsibility of the National Center for Biological Safety and Research (BSRC) to ensure the protection of the public by assessing the safety of chemicals and other materials, as stipulated in the regulations of the NIHS in November 2005. JaCVAM activities are also beneficial to the application and approval for the manufacture and sale of pharmaceutical, chemical, pesticide and other products, as well as to revisions to standards for cosmetic and quasi-drug products [7–9].

Over the past 12 years, JaCVAM has played an active role in gaining approval for the adoption of OECD test guidelines for more than ten different test methods developed by Japanese researchers [6] and has evaluated alternative methods to animal testing based on OECD test guidelines as well as International Conference on Harmonisation of Technical Requirements for Registration of Pharmaceuticals for Human Use (ICH) guidelines. Moreover, JaCVAM has recommended twenty-one test methods for adoption by Japanese regulatory agencies [7], as shown in Table 2. The notification issued by MHLW in 2011 presented JaCVAM with the opportunity to impart a strong impact on testing throughout Japan by accelerating the development of new non-animal test methods.

Guidance for Alternative to Animal Testing

The following guidance documents have been approved by the MHLW [5]. Based on OECD test guidelines and JaCVAM evaluation documents, dermatologists and representatives of cosmetic companies as well as specialists from both the PMDA and the NIHS have drafted guidance documents for a number of alternative test methods.

- Guidance on the use of alternative test methods for skin-sensitization and phototoxicity in safety assessment of cosmetics and quasi-drugs (Appendix 1: Guidance on the use of LLNA[1] for skin sensitisation test as an alternative test method in safety assessments of cosmetics and quasi-drugs, Appendix 2: Guidance on the use of the in vitro 3T3 NRU[2] phototoxicity test as an alternative test method in safety assessments of cosmetics and quasi-drugs), dated April 26, 2012
- Guidance on the use of alternative test methods for skin-sensitization (LLNA:DA, LLNA:BrdU-ELISA) in safety assessments of cosmetics and quasi-drugs, dated May 30, 2013,
- Guidance on the use of the BCOP[3] test as an alternative method for testing ocular irritation in the safety assessment of cosmetics and quasi-drugs, dated February 4, 2014
- Points of consideration for ocular irritation testing in the safety assessment of cosmetics and quasi-drug, dated February 27, 2015
- Guidance on the use of the ICE[4] test as an alternative method for testing ocular irritation in the safety assessment of cosmetics and quasi-drugs, dated November 16, 2015
- Guidance on the use of in vitro skin penetration assay (in vitro skin absorption assay) in the safety assessment of cosmetics and quasi-drugs, dated November 15, 2016
- Guidance on the use of combinations of in vitro skin sensitization assays in the safety assessment of cosmetics and quasi-drugs, dated January 2018.

---

[1] LLNA: Local lymph Node Assay.

[2] NRU: Neutral Red Uptake.

[3] BCOP: Bovine Corneal Opacity and Permeability.

[4] ICE: Isolated Chicken Eye.

Table 2. Test methods proposed to the Ministry of Health, Labour and Welfare by JaCVAM

No.	Test Method
1	*In vitro* skin corrosion testing: i.e. Human Skin Model Test: Vitrolife-Skin, EpiDerm, Episkin, SKinEthics, EpiCS
2	*In vitro* skin corrosion testing: Transcutaneous Electrical Resistance Test Method (TER)
3	*In vitro* skin corrosion testing: *In Vitro* membrane barrier test method for skin corrosion
4	*In vitro* skin irritation testing: i.e. Reconstructed Human Epidermis Test Method, Episkin, Epiderm, SkinEthics and LabCyte EPI-Model
5	Bovine corneal opacity and permeability (BCOP) test for identifying ocular corrosives and severe irritant
6	Isolated chicken eye (ICE) test for identifying ocular corrosives and severe irritants
7	Fluorescein leakage (FL) assay for identifying ocular corrosives and severe irritants
8	Short Time Exposure *In Vitro* Test Method for assessing ocular irritation
9	Reconstructed human Cornea-like Epithelium Eye Irritation Test Method
10	Acute Eye irritation/Corrosion
11	Local lymph node assay (LLNA) and reduced LLNA for identifying skin sensitising substances
12	LLNA:DA, a non-radioactive modification of the LLNA method, which quantifies adenosine triphosphate (ATP) content via bioluminescence, as an indicator of lymphocyte proliferation for identifying skin sensitising substances
13	LLNA:BrdU-enzyme linked immunosorbent assay (ELISA), a non-radioactive modification of the LLNA method, which utilises non-radiolabelled 5-bromo-2-deoxyuridine (BrdU) in an ELISA-based test system, to measure lymphocyte proliferation for identifying skin sensitising substances
14	Direct Peptide Reactivity Assay for skin sensitisation Testing
15	ARE-Nrf2 Luciferase Test Method assay for skin sensitisation testing
16	h-CLAT (human Cell Line Activation Test) for skin sensitisation testing
17	Skin absorption i*n vitro* method
18	Reactive Oxygen Species (ROS) assay for photosafety assessment
19	*In vitro* cytotoxicity test for estimating starting doses for acute oral systemic toxicity tests
20	BG1Luc estrogen receptor transactivation assay (ETRA), for identifying oestrogen receptor agonists and antagonists
21	Stably transfected Transcriptional Activation Assay to Detect ER mediated activity

Almost all Japanese cosmetic companies have stopped animal testing voluntarily and now hope that the MHLW and PMDA will approve the use of new cosmetic ingredients without animal testing. Many procedures for regulatory acceptance still require animal testing, and it is difficult to gain approval even for additives to quasi-drug products without data from animal testing. Given the current situation, JaCVAM has attempted to promote the development of guidance for the use of alternatives to animal testing. Unfortunately, there are still many types of testing for which non-animal test methods are limited. In particular, there are as of yet no suitable non-animal test methods available as alternatives to the LLNA, LLNA:DA, LLNA:BrdU-ELISA, or Draize eye test, and the time has come to accelerate the development of and guidance for the use of in vitro test methods for new cosmetic ingredients.

References

1. EC (2004) Time tables for the phasing-out of animal testing in the framework of the 7th amendment to the cosmetics directive (Council Directive 76/768/EEC). Commission Staff Working Documents, SEC82004)1210
2. MHLW (2011) Guidebook on the manufacture and sales of cosmetics and quasi-drugs [In Japanese]. Yakuji Nippo Ltd, Tokyo, Japan, pp 159–182
3. MHLW (2005) Guide for the care and use of laboratory animals (in Japanese). Ministry of Health, Labour and Welfare, Tokyo, Japan
4. MHLW (2006) Cosmetics standard amendment request and manufacturing and marketing approval of quasi-drugs (in Japanese). Ministry of Health, Labour and Welfare, Tokyo, Japan
5. PMDA (2018) Homepage (in Japanese). Pharmaceuticals and Medical Devices Agency, Tokyo, Japan. https://www.pmda.go.jp/review-services/drug-reviews/about-reviews/q-drugs/0002.html
6. OECD (2018) Test guideline. Organisation for Economic Co-operation and Development, Paris, France. http://www.oecd-ilibrary.org/environment/oecd-guidelines-for-the-testing-of-chemicals-section-4-health-effects_20745788
7. JaCVAM (2018) Homepage. Japanese Center for the Validation of Alternative Methods, Tokyo, Japan. http://www.jacvam.jp/en/index.html
8. Barroso J, Ahn IY, Caldeira C et al (2016) Validation of alternative methods for toxicity testing. Adv Exp Med Biol 856:343–386
9. Kojima H (2013) Update from the Japanese center for the validation of alternative methods (JaCVAM). ATLA 41:435–441

Alternatives and Refinement for Animal Experimentation in Cancer Research

Arvind D. Ingle(✉)

Scientific Officer 'G' & Officer-in-Charge, Laboratory Animal Facility, Tata Memorial Centre, ACTREC, Navi Mumbai 410210, MS, India
aingle@actrec.gov.in

Abstract. Globally cancer is a major public health issue and is a second biggest cause of deaths. Although animal models have limitations in terms of predictive and translational value to humans, they have played a major role in understanding this disease and anticancer drug discovery. In cancer research the most commonly used animal species are mice, rats, hamsters, rabbits, Guinea pigs, fish and amphibians. Use of different cell lines in tissue culture system offers a great relief from use of animals at the same time provide important clues before embarking the animal experiments. Use of spontaneously developing tumor models are encouraged rather producing diseases in the animals. Beside the alternatives, refinement also plays important role in reducing the animal usage in cancer research. However, cancer research use whole body system to evaluate the new strategies for diagnosis and treatment of cancer. This paper highlights the available alternatives and refinements for animal experimentation. A positive note is that if coupled with the refinements, even a minimised number of animal usage shall also yield the meaningful and acceptable results.

Keywords: Cancer research · Animal models · Alternatives · Refinement

Introduction

Cancer researcher plays an important role in investigating new modalities of diagnosis and treatment. This includes discovering the faulty genes and molecules that cause cancer, investigating how the disease grows and spreads, developing and testing new treatment and tests, and exploring how our immune system can help fight tumours. Literature surveys indicate that amongst various species, rodents have been extensively used in biomedical research. The laboratory mouse and rat is a common experimental model, in part because of well-defined strain genealogies, standardized mapping tools, and the availability of sophisticated genetic monitoring technologies. When animals are used for research, it is the moral duty of the scientist to avoid or minimize discomfort, distress, and painful situations. The regulations and policies help to ensure animals are treated humanely. If a procedure involves more than momentary or slight pain or distress, it must be performed using appropriate pain relieving drugs (e.g. sedatives, analgesia or anesthesia) [1].

Knowledge gained through use of animals in research is still improving the life of not only humans but domestic as well as pet and wild animals too. Discovery of

H. Kojima et al. (Eds.): *Alternatives to Animal Testing*, pp. 69–75, 2019.
https://doi.org/10.1007/978-981-13-2447-5_9

antibiotics like penicillin, erythromycin, tetracyclin etc. would have not been possible without involvement of animal testing.

Further the discovery of Nude and SCID mice model have made significant improvement in these models and have made it possible to identify clinically efficacious agents through anticancer research and testing. These models are said to be a '*Workhorse*' of the pharmaceutical industry. These models have not only helped in characterization of cancer cell lines but also helped us in understanding metastatic processes and efficacy of the newly developed anticancer drugs [2].

Cancer researchers need predictive and cost effective preclinical models that more accurately predict the response of human cancer to chemotherapy. Experimental models of human cancers are important in reconstructing the events that occur in human patients with cancers. A variety of factors decides the choice of tumor and model.

Alternatives in Cancer Research

Scientists use many ways to try to replace animals used in research. These include using cell cultures, computer modelling and human studies. Researchers must attempt using these techniques if they would be as effective as using animals.

Responses to chemicals are complex and difficult to accurately assess using only biochemical or cell-based (*in vitro*) systems or computer models. No single *in vitro* test method can be employed to serve all regulatory needs for a specific testing area. Mechanistically based alternative approach may provide promising opportunity for assessing hazards of regulatory concern. Adverse outcome pathways (AOPs) are expected to provide insight into the biological relevance, reliability, and uncertainties associated with the results from *in silico*, *in chemico* and *in vitro* approaches for regulatory use. This provides the biological context and supporting weight of evidence to facilitate the interpretation of such alternative data [3]. Severe eye irritants and substances that could cause allergic contact dermatitis is the only option where major progress has been made in reducing and replacing animal use [4]. For other hazards that can cause cancer or birth defects, development of *in vitro* tests that reliably identify hazards is more difficult because of the number of different mechanisms involved in these complex biological processes. However, some lower vertebrate offers the best alternatives in cancer research.

Zebrafish, *Danio rerio* have become a popular model for studying developmental processes and human diseases. Fish and human solid tumors share a high degree of histological similarity and therefore have been used extensively as model for human cancers. Zebrafish also form spontaneous tumors with similar histopathological and gene expression profile as human tumors [5]. Zebrafish have proved to be useful for use in cancer research over the last decade. There are several long-standing methods for establishing a cancer model in zebrafish, including carcinogenic treatment, transgenic regulation, and the transplantation of mammalian tumor cells. Some of the analysis of metastasis pathway is conducted in tightly controlled *in vitro* cell system usually involving up-regulation or down-regulation of genes. These assays include trans-well motility, wound healing, invasion and hanging drop assays. These assays do not answer issues of intravasation of tumor cells into blood vessels or extravasation in to distant organs. In order to study these processes, there is no alternative to *in vivo* systems. However, zebrafish can offer these assays as an alternative to rodents or other vertebrates animals to study the human tumor angiogenesis or metastasis. Because of the transparent in nature, Zebrafish offer excellent features to study tumor angiogenesis as well as metastasis [6, 7]. Reports have also shown that primary human cancer cells can metastasize in fish and this ability can be used to predict metastatic potential in a clinical setting. Zebrafish has been used to study the metastasis of lymphoblastic leukemia, melanoma, breast tumor, prostate cancer, rhabdomyosarcoma, testicular cancer, colon cancer, neuroblastoma and pancreatic tumors [8–13].

Organisms like Hydra have been used as a model for regeneration, embryogenesis, testing the water pollutant eco-pollutant and environmental genomics [14, 15]. However, it remains to be seen whether they can also be used explored for studying the carcinogenesis.

Efforts are also targeted towards use of 'artificial tumor' tissue grown from stem cells or a combination of tumor cells and tumor stromal cells etc. [16, 17]. Full-thickness skin models can be used to test the effect of substance in question on the skin tissues. However, since cancer research needs a complete body system for testing, this model may be of little hopes.

Use of spontaneously developing tumor models like leukemia, lung cancer, brain cancer and breast cancer caused by MMTV or any other aetiology are encouraged in lieu of producing these diseases in the animals.

3R's

WMS Russell and RL Burch originated the concepts of replacement, reduction, and refinement, which they published in their book in 1959 entitled "*The Principles of Humane Experimental Technique*" [18]. Russell and Burch proposed that if animals were to be used in experiments, every effort should be made to 'Replace' them with non-sentient alternatives, to 'Reduce' to a minimum number of animals used, and to 'Refine' the experiments so that they caused the minimum pain and distress.

Replacement alternatives advocate methods to be used in achieving scientific results without conducting experiments on animals. There is a direct correlation between larger number of animals used to higher overall costs and animal suffering. Therefore, the number of animals used should be kept to a minimum that would be consistent with the research objectives. Refinement alternatives include methods that alleviate or minimize potential pain and distress thus emphasizing on animal well-being.

CPCSEA

The Institutional Animal Care and Use Committee (IACUC) or Institutional Animal Ethics Committee (IAEC) is legally required to oversee all animal care and use activities conducted at their institution. IACUC/IAEC is also required to set high ethical and welfare standards for using the animals. In India the Committee for the Purpose of Control and Supervision of Experiments on Animals (CPCSEA), established under the Ministry of Environment, Forests and Climate Change has been instrumental in avoiding the animal usage or if not possible, to reduce the number of animals used in experimentation. At the local level, IACUC/IAEC are mandated to ensure that: the number of animals used for the research in each groups are enough to yield statistically valid results; appropriate species of animal is used for the project; humane experimental endpoints have been established and appropriate methods of euthanasia are being utilized [19]. The CPCSEA integrate the 3R's in all R&D processes and procedures. It gives emphasis on review of animal models on a continuous basis for replacement with alternatives. It also promotes use of human cells and tissues instead of living animals, wherever possible. The CPCSEA is charged with reviewing and approving all research and testing activities in India that involve animals before scientists begin their experiments to ensure that there are no alternatives to using animals, that research is not being unnecessarily duplicated, and the experiment is relevant to human or animal health and will be for the betterment of the society.

Refinement in Cancer Research

For more than a half century mice have been the primary species in which experimental cancer chemotherapy have been tested [20]. Cancer drug screening program of the US National Cancer Institute (NCI) started with the ascitic and then with solid tumors. This program used conventional mouse models like C57BL/6, Swiss, BALB/c and DBA/2 strains. After the discovery of the Nude and SCID mice, widespread use of human tumor transplantation for anticancer research and testing was made possible [21, 22]. Mice and rats often develop benign and malignant cancers spontaneously. The incidence may vary from strain to strain. These spontaneous tumors do not always metastasize to different organs or have mild local tissue invasion and therefore the incidence is very rare. However, majority of the data generated on the metastatic behavior of cancer is reported to be derived from studies in rodent models only [23, 24].

'Specialized' models like transgenic, knock out, Nude, SCID and hairless SCID mouse models have played a central role in cancer research. Models like SCID beige, NIH-III, NOD-SCID, SCID beige, NSG, NOG and Rag-1 and 2 mutation mouse model which lack T-, B- as well as NK cell activity are the next level of 'super specialized' models, which supports not only the hetero-transplantation but also the metastasis studies.

Use of T- and B-cell deficient animals as shown by the use of flow cytometry; use of rodent pathogen-free animals; use of genetically proven animal models; use of appropriate number of cells and volume for injection; use of appropriate route of injection; and use of properly genotyped/phenotyped animal models helps to reduce the number of animals used for the respective research and also yield authentic and reproducible results. Use of spontaneously developing tumor models such as mammary gland tumors in C3H/J mice, leukemia in AKR mice, lung cancer in A/J mice and brain tumor in *Ptch* or *Smo* knockout mice is one of the refinements. New tumors or tumor-like growth found in the laboratory animals can be a potential material to study the disease processes. Spontaneously developing papilloma incidence has been reported in Nude mice by Ingle et al., 2011 [25]. These are characterized to be caused by mouse papillomaviruses. This model has been exploited and characterized fully for its cause, genomic analysis, molecular diagnosis and sequencing of the virus. [26–29].

In order to ascertain the absence of T- and B-cells in the immune-compromised animals, assessment of these cells by flow cytometry is the best method [30]. This can be done by measuring the CD3 antibodies for T-cells and CD19 antibodies for B-cells. Additionally, subsets of CD3 can also be checked by including CD4 and CD8 antibodies.

Conclusion

Use of animals remains unavoidable for the time being for the development of new and more effective methods for diagnosis and treating diseases that affect both humans and animals. However, it is our moral duty to see that the use of animals is either replaced or atleast minimized to the extent to get the meaningful as well as reproducible and acceptable results. With its own advantages and disadvantages, the zebrafish embryo as well as zebrafish tumor xenograft model can be very well used as a tool for investigating the cancer biology including neovascularization for drug discovery and gene targeting in tumor angiogenesis. With refinement of the quality of animals through genetic & microbiological testing, refining the volume and route of injection and use of spontaneously available tumor models, it is possible to achieve the same results in cancer research.

References

1. DeHaven WR (2000) Pain and distress: USDA Perspective Definition of pain and distress and reporting requirements for laboratory animals. In: Proceedings of the Workshop held June 22, 2000, National Academy Press, Washington, D.C, pp 9–12
2. Morton CL, Houghton PJ (2007) Establishment of human tumor xenografts in immunodeficient mice. Nat Protoc 2:247–250
3. Tollefsen KE et al (2014) Applying adverse outcome pathway (AOPs) to support integrated approaches to testing and assessment (IATA). Reg Toxicol Pharmacol 70(3):629–640
4. Westmoreland C, Holmes AM (2009) Assuring consumer safety without animals. Organogenesis 5(2):67–72
5. Zhao S, Huang J, Ye J (2015) A fresh look at zebrafish from the perspective of cancer research. J Exp Clin Cancer Res 34:80
6. Tobia C, De Sena G, Presta M (2011) Zebrafish embryo, a tool to study tumor angiogenesis. Int J Dev Biol 55:505–509
7. Tobia C et al (2013) Zebrafish embryo as a tool to study tumor/endothelial cell cross-talk. Biochem Biophys Acta 1832:1371–1377

8. Feitsma H, Cuppen E (2008) Zebra fish as cancer model. Mol Cancer Res 6(5):685–694
9. Taylor AM, Zon LI (2009) Zebrafish tumor assays: the state of transplantation. Zebrafish. 6 (4):339–346
10. Mione MC, Trede NS (2010) The zebrafish as a model for cancer. Dis Model Mech. 3(9–10):517–523
11. Teng Y et al (2013) Evaluating human cancer cell metastasis in Zebra fish. BMC Cancer 13:453
12. Yang X et al (2013) A novel zebrafish xenotransplantation model for study of glioma stem cell invasion. PLoS ONE 8(4):e61801. https://doi.org/10.1371/journal.pone.0061801
13. Kanungo J et al (2014) Zebra fish model in drug safety assessment. Curr Pharm Des 20 (34):5416–5429
14. Gierer A (2012) The Hydra model- a model for what? Int J Dev Biol 56:437–445
15. Murugadas A (2016) Hydra as a model organism to decipher the toxic effects of copper oxide nanorod: Eco-toxicogenomics approach. Sci Rep 15(6):29663. https://doi.org/10.1038/srep29663
16. Kammerer R, von Kleist S (1995) Artificial tumor: a three dimensional in vitro model of individual human solid tumors. Tumour Biol 16(4):213–221
17. Lyden T, Martin M (2016) Modelling melanoma as in vitro artificial tumor tissue using natural 3D matrix material. FASEB 30(1):697–81
18. Russel WMS, Rex LB (1959) The principles of humane experimental technique, Methuen & Co. London, Special edition published by Universities Federation for Animal Welfare (UFAW), 1992
19. Standard Operating Procedure for Institutional Animal Ethics Committee, CPCSEA (2010) Min. of Environment & Forests, Govt. of India, January 2010, pp 11–14. http://cpcsea.nic.in/Content/55_1_PUBLICATIONS.aspx
20. Kerbel RS (2003). Human tumor xenograft as predictive preclinical model for anticancer drug activity in humans. Cancer Biol Ther. 2 (4–1): S 134–139
21. Johnson JI, Decker S, Zaharevitz D et al (2003) Relationship between drug activity in NCI preclinical in vitro and in vivo model and early clinical trials. Br J Cancer 9:1424–1431
22. Sausville EA, Burger AM (2006) Contributions of human tumor xenograft to anticancer drug development. Cancer Res 66(7):3351–3354
23. Giavazzi R, Campbell DE, Jessup JM et al (1986) Metastatic behaviour of tumor cells isolated form primary and metastatic humnan colorectal carcinomas implanted into different sites in Nude mice. Cancer Res 46:1929–1933
24. Morikawa K, Walker SM, Jessup JM et al (1988) In vivo selction of highly metastatic cells from surgical specimens of different primary human colon carcinomas implanted into Nude mice. Cancer Res 48:1943–1948
25. Ingle A et al (2011) Novel laboratory mouse papillomavirus (MusPV) infection. Vet Pathol 48(2):500–505
26. Joh J et al (2011) Genomic analysis of the only known laboratory mouse papillomavirus (MusPV). J Gen Virol 92:692–698
27. Joh J et al (2012) Molecular diagnosis of a laboratory mouse papillomavirus (MusPV). Exp Mol Pathol 93(3): 416–421 (Dec. 2012)
28. Sundberg JP et al (2014) Immune status, strain background, and anatomic site of innoculation affect mouse papillomavirus (MmuPV1) induction of exophytic papillomas or endophytic trichoblastomas. PLoS ONE 9(12):1–28

29. Joh J et al (2014) Searching for the initiating site of the major capsid protein to generate virus-like particles for a novel laboratory mouse papillomavirus. Exp Mol Pathol 96(2): 155–161
30. Thorat R, Ahire S, Ingle A (2013) Re-establishment of breeding colony of NOD SCID mice from revival of cryo-preserved embryos. Lab Anim 42(4):131–134

3Rs in Quality Control of Human Vaccines: Opportunities and Barriers

Sylvie Uhlrich[1(✉)], Emmanuelle Coppens[1], Frederic Moysan[1], Sue Nelson[2], and Nolwenn Nougarede[1]

[1] Sanofi Pasteur, Marcy L'Etoile, France
Sylvie.uhlrich@sanofi.com
[2] Sanofi Pasteur, Toronto, Canada

Abstract. The 3Rs principles – Replacement, Reduction, Refinement – were established in 1959 and since then have been adopted widely and particularly in Europe with the European Directive 2010/63/EU. The vaccine industry in Europe has been committed to the 3Rs principles for several years, including animal welfare as well as for reducing and replacing animal use in research, non-clinical safety and analytical testing.

Whereas animal testing has been successfully removed from lot release testing of well-characterized human vaccines, large numbers of laboratory animals continue to be used for safety and potency quality control testing for established inactivated vaccines such as rabies, pertussis, diphtheria, and tetanus vaccines.

Moreover, specifications for human vaccine batch approval often differ between various parts of the world, resulting in either duplication of animal testing or partial implementation of 3Rs for some vaccines when distributed worldwide. This reinforces the need for enhancing international harmonization and cooperation efforts.

In this chapter, we review the use of laboratory animals in human vaccines research and quality control and describe the vaccine manufacturing industry commitments and its concrete programs for implementing 3Rs principles in R&D and industrial operations processes. We highlight the successes as well as the barriers that are encountered when implementing 3Rs principles, as well as the ongoing efforts that include international collaborations with other industries, public organizations and Health Authorities for the acceptance of alternative methods.

Animal Use in Vaccine Quality Control

Vaccine quality control tests have their roots in the 19th century with the work of L. Pasteur, R. Koch, E. von Behring, P. Ehrlich and others. Test design based on multi-dilutions assays and using a reference preparation in parallel to the vaccine to be tested was introduced in the 30–50 s of past century by Prigge [1]. The current *in vivo* quality control tests have been developed in the 50 s–70 s of the previous century (for example: the Kendrick test for Pertussis vaccine, the NIH test for Rabies vaccine). A sharp increase in animal numbers used for vaccine quality control has been observed since the 50 s.

H. Kojima et al. (Eds.): *Alternatives to Animal Testing*, pp. 76–82, 2019.
https://doi.org/10.1007/978-981-13-2447-5_10

Today, testing of biologicals has the highest proportion of experiments causing severe pain and distress to animals out of various types of experiments (basic research, non-clinical testing, and quality control). The vaccine industry accounts for a high proportion of these animals. Animals are used for vaccine development (research, non-clinical evaluation of safety & efficacy), production as well as batch control testing for safety and potency. Vaccines quality control is responsible for the vast majority of animal used by vaccine manufacturers. Moreover, in addition to animals used for batch control testing by vaccine manufacturers, there are additional animals used by National Control Laboratories when duplicating some of the control tests.

3Rs History and Vaccine Context

The principles of Humane Experimental Technique were first described by William Russel and Rex Burch in 1959 [2]. An important step in international coordination of 3Rs efforts for vaccines quality control was achieved at the conference organized by IABS in London in 1985. The concept of 3Rs in vaccine research and testing translates as follows:

- **Replacement** means implementing methods which avoid or replace the use of animals
- **Reduction**, means changing the test design in order to minimize the number of animals per experiment
- **Refinement**: means moving to methods that minimize suffering and improve animal welfare (e.g. replacing challenge tests by immunogenicity assays)

There are four main drivers that justify implementing 3Rs in vaccine quality control.

The first driver is animal welfare: Animals are sentient beings, large number of animals is used for vaccine quality control and a large proportion of those animals are exposed to severe pain and distress, and there is a growing societal concern regarding the use of animals for scientific purposes.

The second driver is Science: *In vivo* models act as a black box and their relevance to human is sometimes questionable; they often show poor robustness and high variability inherent to the use of live individuals. The technologies and the scientific knowledge have evolved over the past years and state of the art *in vitro* technologies are now more performant and relevant than animal *in vivo* assay to evaluate the consistency of a vaccine.

The third driver is Economics*: In vivo* tests are time consuming and human resource demanding; *in vivo* tests are expensive due to the animals themselves, and have long cycle times (several weeks for most *in vivo* potency assays as well as some safety tests). Moreover, the high variability can lead to rejection of safe and efficacious vaccines, thus inducing delays to market release and vaccine shortages.

The fourth driver is the regulatory context: 3Rs have now become legal requirement in Europe; it started with EMA guidance in 1997 [3], followed by a first directive in 2001 for medicinal as well as veterinary products [4]. The key directive on the protection of animals used for scientific purposes was issued in June 2010 [5] with the following statement: "Member States shall ensure that, wherever possible, a scientifically satisfactory method or testing strategy, not entailing the use of live animals, shall be used…"

In addition, the 3Rs offer an opportunity for harmonization. There is today no worldwide harmonized framework, leading to many divergent local regulatory requirements. As a vaccine may be registered in more than 100 countries for which there are different release requirements, this translates into having to apply various *in vivo* methods for one product, which leads to additional complexity for supply chain, for testing and regulatory submissions, as well as more animals used per batch release (in practice we may end up with 4 repeat testing between manufacturer and the different National Control Laboratories involved in batch release). The ultimate impact is increased costs and timelines with no added value on the quality of the product, a risk of vaccine shortage, and finally a negative impact on public health.

3Rs Successes

Table 1 presents the current status for the use of alternative methods, in the European Pharmacopeia and in vaccine industry respectively.

For all vaccines, the European Pharmacopeia has waived the General Safety Test from routine testing. In practice, this test is omitted for all new vaccines, but not yet for all existing vaccines due to local requirements, as well as time needed to submit variations in all countries.

For the test for specific toxicity for diphtheria vaccines, the European Pharmacopeia allows performing a cell-based method at Drug Substance stage, and to waive the test at Drug Product stage, and this is partially implemented again due to local requirements.

For the test for specific toxicity for Pertussis vaccines, the European Pharmacopeia allows performing a cell-based method at Drug Substance stage, and this is partially implemented depending on the product; applying the cell-based assay as well as omitting the test at Drug Product stage is under evaluation at European Pharmacopeia.

For oral Polio vaccine neurovirulence test, switching from non-human primates to transgenic mice is described in European Pharmacopeia and implemented. For inactivated Polio vaccine (IPV) inactivation test, the European Pharmacopeia allows replacing the primary monkey kidney; the L20B cell line is routinely used.

For testing of adventitious agents, the removal of tests on guinea pigs and eggs is applicable in European Pharmacopeia since January 2017, and the implementation is ongoing. Moreover, the replacement of *in vivo* tests by broad molecular methods is described in European Pharmacopeia since January 2017, and developments to support implementation are ongoing.

For potency assay for diphtheria and tetanus vaccines, the European Pharmacopeia allows using serological instead of lethal endpoints, and allows moving to single dilution assays and this is partially implemented, depending on product and market.

For IPV, the European Pharmacopeia allows replacing the *in vivo* assay by an immunochemical assay (ELISA), and this is implemented for most products but not all due to local requirements.

Table 1. Use of alternative methods to *in vivo* safety and potency tests for vaccines

Possible use of alternative methods	Ph. Eur.	Vaccine industry
All vaccines Allow omission of abnormal toxicity test / general safety test	☒	☒ partial
Specific Toxicity test for Diphtheria vaccines Allow the use of a VERO cell-based method at DS* Remove the test at DP**	 ☒ ☒	 ☒partial ☒partial
Specific Toxicity test for Pertussis vaccines Allow CHO cell-based assay to replace HIST : at DS* at DP** stage	 ☒ ongoing	 ☒partial Devt
Neurovirulence Test for Oral Polio Vaccine Allow switch from non-human primate to transgenic mice	☒	☒
Inactivation test for inactivated Polio Vaccine Allow replacement of 1ry monkey kidney cells with L20B cell line	☒	☒partial
Test for adventitious agents Removal of GP & embryonated eggs for cell bank testing Replace *in vivo* tests by broad molecular methods (HTS***)	 ☒ ☒	 ☒ongoing ☒Devt
Potency tests for D and T vaccines • Allow using serology instead of lethal endpoints • Allow introducing single-dilution assay	 ☒ ☒	 ☒partial ☒partial
Potency test for inactivated Polio Vaccine Allow *in vitro* test	☒	☒partial
Potency test for inactivated Rabies Vaccine Allow *in vitro* test	☒	☒Devt
Potency test for inactivated Hepatitis A vaccine Allow *in vitro* test	☒	☒
Potency test for inactivated Hepatitis B vaccine Allow *in vitro* test	☒	☒
Potency test for Haemophilus influenzae vaccine Allow *in vitro* test	☒	☒
Potency test for human Papilloma vaccine Allow *in vitro* test	☒	☒

(*) DS : Drug Substance
(**) DP: Drug Product
(***) HTS: High Throughput Sequencing

For the potency assay for inactivated rabies vaccines, the European Pharmacopeia allows using an immunochemical method and such assay has been developed at Sanofi Pasteur [6] and is under validation in the frame of an international working group [7].

For the potency assays for hepatitis A and B respectively, haemophilus Influenzae and human papilloma vaccines, the European Pharmacopeia allows using immunochemical methods and this is implemented for both vaccines.

Barriers to 3Rs

There are two main barriers to 3Rs implementation: one is regulatory and the other is scientific.

The main regulatory hurdles are:

- the lack of harmonization of regulatory requirements, worldwide
- the prudence of health authorities to accept deviations from established guidelines
- the complexity of regulatory changes that discourage and slow development and implementation of alternatives to animal testing; this is one of the main reasons why industry has not been able to fully implement alternative tests described in European Pharmacopeia.

The key scientific hurdles are:

- The inherent variability of *in vivo* assays
- The fact that the *in vivo* assays are not validated as per ICH requirements [8]
- The fact that the product quality attributes will likely be assessed differently when changing from an *in vivo* to an *in vitro* method.

Therefore, a one-to-one comparison is often challenging and not necessarily justified.

Perspectives for the Future

This is the time for moving from the concept of test replacement to the concept of test substitution that is based on demonstrating the scientific relevance of the new test.

For potency tests, this means demonstrating the capability of new test to control key quality attributes and maintain link with batches found efficacious through clinical studies or through routine use as well as the capability of the *in vitro* test to detect differences that are relevant to the control of the production process.

For safety tests, the *in vitro* method should be specific and at least as sensitive as *in vivo* assay. Where possible, a functional assay should be used; otherwise, the alternative method should be based on the detection of parameter(s) reflecting the mode of action of the toxic component.

Moving from one-to-one replacement or substitution to an integrated approach aims at implementing the "consistency approach" that was described by de Mattia et al. in 2011 [9] and is based on the strict application of GMP rules and guidelines, process validation, in process and final product tests, and is aimed at verifying that a manufacturing process produces final batches which are consistent with one that fulfils all the criteria of Quality, Safety and Efficacy as defined in the marketing authorization, ultimately resulting in replacement of routinely used *in vivo* tests.

Concluding Remarks

3Rs acceptability is based on full implementation of GMP, reliable, standardized and validated processes, in process monitoring, consistent product demonstrated safe & efficacious, relevant science and validated tests (as per ICH Q2(R1)).

Regulatory acceptance of 3Rs is easier for new vaccines. For existing vaccines, manufacturers need help in order to facilitate post-approval changes based on:

- a mutual understanding, recognition and implementation of the change by all stakeholders in a timely manner
- a global harmonization of regulatory requirements endorsed by an international organization
- involvement of all stakeholders (regulators, scientists, animal welfare organizations, the public and decision makers) for communication of best practices.

International collaboration is a key element for the implementation of 3Rs principles and the European vaccine industry is involved in several international projects or working groups such as:

- European Partnership for Alternative to Animals (EPAA) and more specifically in a project dedicated to the replacement of NIH potency assay for human Rabies Vaccine [7] as well as in another project working on harmonization of 3Rs in Biologicals which is currently focusing on the deletion of GST worldwide [10]
- An international working group sponsored by NIH, ICCVAM, NC3Rs and EDQM that has been working on the replacement of the histamine test for Pertussis specific toxicity at Drug Product stage from 2010–2015, that may lead to the introduction of a cell-based method in European Pharmacopeia
- The Vac2Vac project which is supported by the European Innovative Medicines initiative (IMI), which is a public-private partnership between the European Union and the European Federation of Pharmaceutical Industries and Associations (EFPIA). Vac2Vac is a 5-year project with a total budget around 16 M euros, and involves 21 partners, 15 public, 6 vaccines manufacturers, from veterinary and human vaccine industries. The objective of the project is to provide the proof of concept to support use of the "consistency approach" for quality control of established vaccines using sets (toolbox) of *in vitro* analytical methods.

References

1. Prigge R (1955) The development of diphtheria vaccines. Bull World Health Organ 13 (3):473–478. The 3Rs principles—Replacement, Reduction, Refinement—have been established
2. Russell WMS, Burch RL (1959) The principles of humane experimental technique. London, UK. Methuen. Reprinted by UFAW: 8 Hamilton Close, South Mimms, Potters Bar, Herts EN6 3QD England, 1992
3. EMA/CPMP/SWP/728/95 (adopted 1997): Replacement of animal studies by *in vitro* models

4. Directive 2001/83/EC of the European parliament and of the council of 6 November 2001 on the 66 Community code relating to medicinal products for human use (Consolidated version: 67 05/10/2009); 68
5. Directive 2010/63/EU of the European parliament and of the council of 22 September 2010 on the protection of animals used for scientific purposes. Text with EEA relevance
6. Chabaud-Riou M et al (2017) Rabies SP G-protein based ELISA as a potency test for rabies vaccines, Biologicals
7. Morgeaux S et al (2017) Replacement of *in vivo* human rabies vaccine potency testing by *in vitro* glycoprotein quantification using ELISA—results of an international collaborative study. Vaccine 35:966–971
8. ICH Harmonized Tripartite Guideline Q2(R1), November 2005, Validation of analytical procedures text and methodology
9. De Mattia F et al (2011) The consistency approach for quality control of vaccines—a strategy to improve quality control and implement 3Rs. Biologicals 39:59–65
10. Schutte K et al (2017) Modern science for better quality control of medicinal products towards global harmonization of 3Rs in biologicals: the report of an EPAA workshop. Biologicals 48:55–65

The Use of Adverse Outcome Pathways (AOPs) to Support Chemical Safety Decisions Within the Context of Integrated Approaches to Testing and Assessment (IATA)

Catherine Willett(✉)

Animal Research Issues, Humane Society of the United States/Humane Society International, 1255 23rd Street NW, Suite 450, Washington, D.C. 20037, USA
kwillett@humanesociety.org

Abstract. New streamlined approaches that use fewer resources and animals are needed for the safety assessment of chemicals. Data gathering should be streamlined to fit regulatory need and the specific properties of the chemicals being assessed. Toward this goal, the Organization for Economic Cooperation and Development (OECD) has introduced the concept of integrated approaches to testing and assessment (IATA) to inform hazard or risk assessment. An IATA is designed to address a specific question, and may include exposure or regulatory considerations, depending on the context. IATA can be informed by mechanistic information about the chemical and related biology. OECD's of Adverse Outcome Pathways (AOPs) framework is designed to gather biological information related to adverse outcomes of regulatory significance. An AOP is the collected chemical and biological information about a particular biological pathway. The OECD has developed guidance for building and assessing AOPs, and is coordinating development of the AOP Knowledge-base (AOP-KB) for collecting and using this information. The AOP-KB also accepts information about the perturbations of these pathways caused by chemical exposure – information can be used to design prediction models. AOPs can form the logical basis for the integration of information and the design of integrated testing strategies (ITS), within the context of an (IATA), to more effectively and efficiently inform hazard or risk determination.

Keywords: Adverse Outcome Pathway (AOP) · Integrated Approach to Testing and Assessment (IATA) · Chemical safety assessment
New Approach Methodologies (NAM)

Introduction

There are scientific, social, economic, practical and regulatory pressures stimulating the development and use of streamlined chemical testing and assessment approaches, including increased reliance on non-animal approaches [also called new approach methodologies (NAM)]. Advances in biological understanding as well as in experimental technologies (e.g. 'omics tools, cell culturing, reconstructed tissues) have allowed the consideration of dramatically different approaches to chemical safety

H. Kojima et al. (Eds.): *Alternatives to Animal Testing*, pp. 83–90, 2019.
https://doi.org/10.1007/978-981-13-2447-5_11

assessment than those traditionally practiced. Increasingly, combinations of non-testing and non-animal test methods are replacing apical animal tests.

For example, there are perhaps tens of thousands of industrial chemicals already in use and in the environment about which there is little toxicological information, and many new chemicals are developed each year, necessitating implementation of a new approach that can broadly assess a large number of chemicals relatively quickly. Another driver comes from the personal care product sector where consumers and regional laws are increasing pressure to develop products without testing on animals. To build a more efficient process, a 2007 National Research Council (NRC) report recommends "Transform(ing) toxicity testing from a system based on whole animal testing to one founded primarily on *in vitro* methods that evaluate changes in biologic processes using cell, cell lines, or cellular components, preferably of human origin" (NRC 2007).

The Adverse Outcome Pathway (AOP) Framework

In order to be able to make decisions using this new type of information, we need to understand how changes at the molecular level in cells and tissues are related to the apical adverse outcomes (such as tumor development, changes in organ size or histology, or death) that toxicologists are more familiar with Fig. 1). The Organization of Economic Cooperation and Development (OECD) has created the Adverse Outcome Pathway framework to collect, organize and evaluate the biological information that links upstream molecular changes with downstream organ, organism and population changes (Fig. 1). According the OECD AOP handbook, AOPs "can be viewed as a sequence of events commencing with initial interactions of a stressor with a biomolecule in a target cell or tissue (i.e., molecular initiating event), progressing through a dependent series of intermediate events and culminating with an adverse outcome… AOPs are typically represented sequentially, moving from one key event to another, as compensatory mechanisms and feedback loops are overcome" (OECD 2018).

Every AOP consists of a variable number and arrangement of a few key elements: a molecular initiating event (MIE), the adverse outcome (AO) of regulatory relevance, any number of intermediate Key Events (KE) and the relationships between these elements (key event relationships or KERs). Five general principles are involved in AOP development: (1) AOPs are not chemical specific, (2) AOPs are modular (consisting of KEs and KERs) that can be shared between two or more pathways, (3) An individual AOP is a pragmatic unit of development and evaluation; (4) for most real-world applications, AOP networks are the functional unit of prediction, and (5) AOPs are living documents, and, as more information is discovered, will be continuously updated and never really finished (Villeneuve et al. 2014). OECD is coordinating the development of the software (the AOP knowledge-base or AOP-KB) as well as a number of guidance documents to facilitate the development, evaluation and use of AOPs. In addition, the Human Toxicology Project Consortium (which is coordinated by the Humane Society of the United States), in collaboration with OECD's AOP program, has created a training course that is freely available to anyone. These

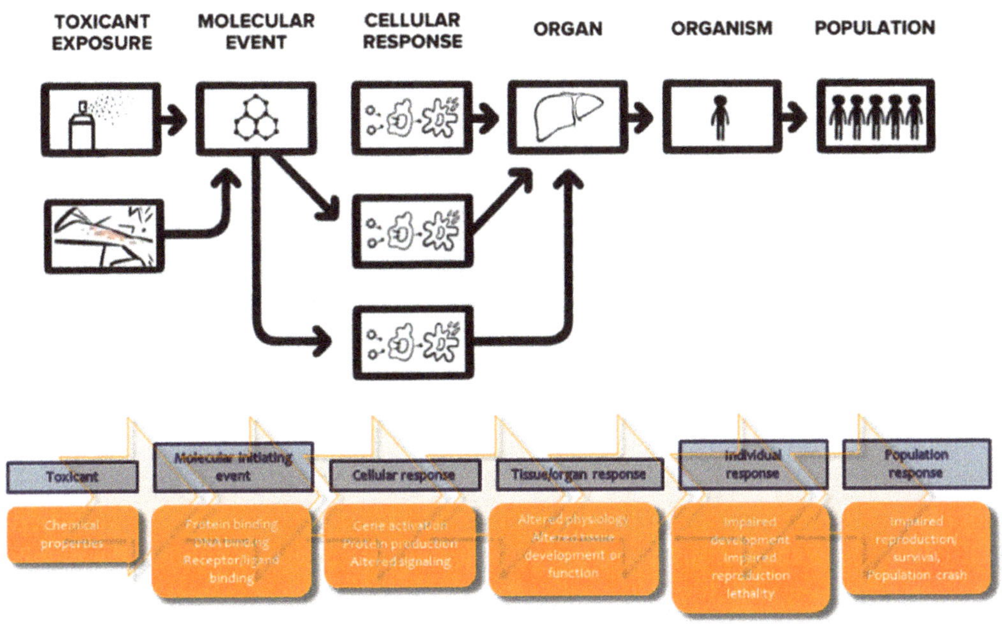

Fig. 1. Linking upstream molecular changes to adverse outcomes: the Adverse Outcome Pathway (AOP) project of the Organization for Economic Cooperation and Development (OECD). (Diagram from "Pathways to a Better Future" video series, © The Human Toxicology Project Consortium).

documents are available from the OECD website, and the training course is available from the HTPC website or at https://aopwiki.org.[1]

The main element of the AOP-KB is currently the AOP Wiki (https://aopwiki.org). The AOP wiki is designed to capture all of the information about AOP elements in text form, via standardized drop-down menus (to keep a standard format and consistent ontology) and free text fields (to accommodate data, explanations and references). As of this writing, there are more than 200 AOPs and more than 1000 KEs and KERs described in the wiki linked to 340 different stressors (metrics available on the AOP Wiki). As more pathways are described, connections between KEs that are common to different pathways are identified, and in this way, biological networks, which are the basis for predicting AOs from MIEs, are discovered.

The AOP Wiki also supports evaluation of the consistency, quantity and quality of the information supporting the KERs and AOP overall (Table 1). The criteria for evaluating KERs and AOPs, modified from the Bradford-Hill criteria for evaluating causal linkages are described in the OECD guidance and in Meek et al. 2014. AOPs that are published in the OECD program series are evaluated in two stages. The first review is by members of the OECD AOP program to make sure the information has been entered in compliance with OECD guidance. The second stage is an independent scientific review by a subject matter expert group that can be a combination of OECD

[1] OECD AOP Program: http://www.oecd.org/chemicalsafety/testing/adverse-outcome-pathways-molecular-screening-and-toxicogenomics.htm; HTPC training course: https://humantoxicologyproject.org/about-pathways-2/aop-online-course/.

Table 1. Biological plausibility: between KE upstream and KE downstream?

High (strong): Extensive understanding of KER	Moderate: KER is plausible	Low (weak): some empirical support
Essentiality: are downstream KEs prevented if upstream KE's blocked?		
High (strong): direct evidence from experimental studies	Moderate: indirect evidence	Low (weak) No or contradictory evidence
Empirical Evidence: amount, quality, consistent, inconsistent?		
High (strong): extensive evidence for temporal, dose-response	Moderate: multiple reports of consistent evidence, some inconsistent	Low (weak): limited or no studies and/or significant inconsistencies

Extracted from OECD (2018), Annex I.

and outside experts - this is similar to peer review of a scientific publication. Once the authors and reviewers are satisfied, a "snapshot" of the AOP at that time is published on the OECD website and is considered the current state of knowledge about that pathway.

The Use of AOPs to Support Hazard and Risk Assessment

The AOP framework has been developed to facilitate the use of molecular and cell-based information to inform regulatory decisions. AOPs on their own are nothing more than organized and, in some cases, evaluated information; however, they can be used in several different ways to support chemical assessment. For example, AOPs can be used to support weight-of-evidence (WoE) evaluation of new or existing information (as is current performed during hazard and risk evaluations), they can be used to generate hypothesis to develop new information for answering a specific regulatory question (as in the context of an integrated approach to testing and assessment, IATA, described in more detail below), or if enough quantitative information is available, they can be used to create predictive models.

To streamline AOP-supported chemical assessment, OECD has also provided guidance for developing and assessing IATA.[2] OECD guidance on developing IATA defines IATA as "pragmatic, science-based approaches for chemical hazard or risk characterization that rely on an *integrated analysis of existing information in a weight of evidence assessment coupled with the generation of new information using testing strategies*…IATA follow an iterative approach to answer a defined question in a specific regulatory context…" (Sachana and Leinala 2017; OECD 2016b). The IATA framework is flexible and allows streamlining of the testing and assessment process to generate exactly the information needed to make a decision. IATA can be as simple or as complex as needed to answer the specific question, depending on the amount of certainty needed.

AOPs can support IATA development and implementation in a number of ways (Fig. 2). AOPs can support WoE evaluation of existing data and, in cases where more

[2] OECD Integrated Approaches to Testing and Assessment: http://www.oecd.org/chemicalsafety/risk-assessment/iata-integrated-approaches-to-testing-and-assessment.htm.

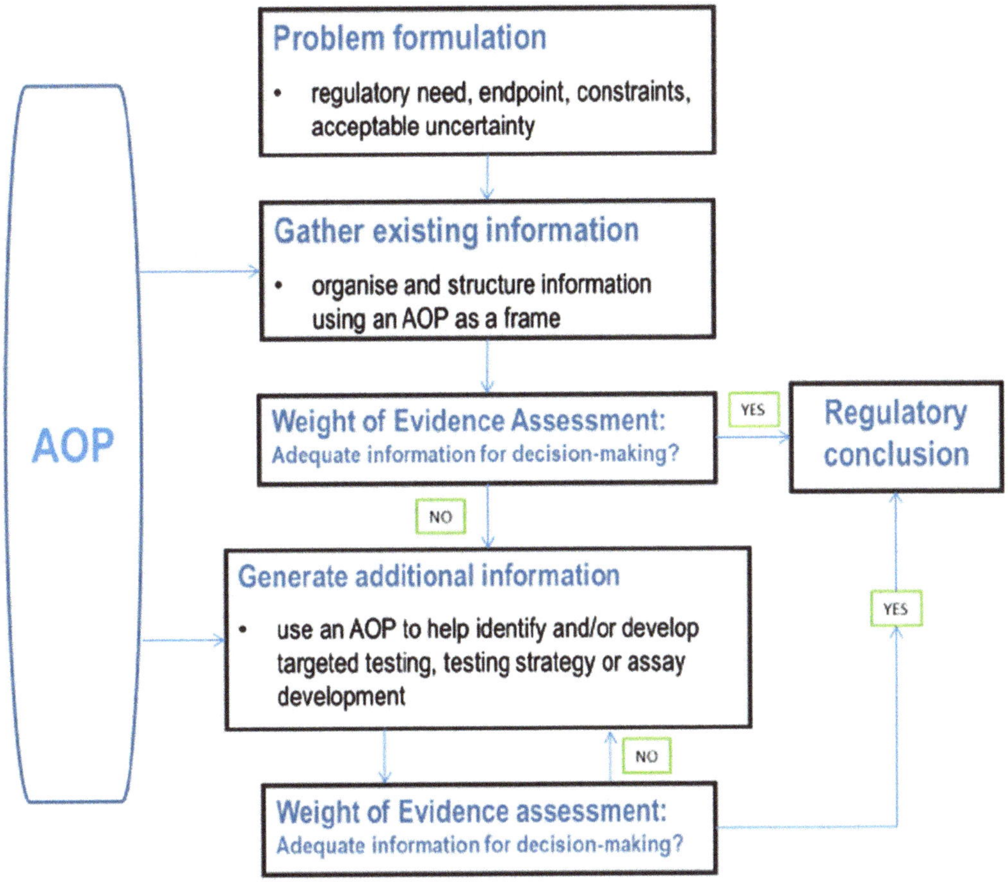

Fig. 2. AOPs can support Integrated Approaches to Testing and Assessment (IATA). (Diagram reprinted from OECD (2016a).

information is needed, identify what information would decrease uncertainty and suggest the method by which to obtain that information. AOPs can be consulted iteratively until sufficient information is obtained to answer the question with the required certainty.

While IATA are designed to be flexible, tailored approaches to address regulatory needs, the potential variability in IATA can cause uncertainty for regulators as well as the regulated community. If there are several different ways to answer the same regulatory question, how do regulators know that each are equally reliable, and how can the submitters of the data be assured of regulatory acceptance? To address this potential regulatory issue, individual standardized IATA, with defined methods and interpretation procedures can be evaluated for regulatory application. OECD has published guidance to facilitate standardization and evaluation of IATA (OECD 2016b). According to this guidance, there are six general principles that are included in every IATA: the defined approach should be associated with the following set of information: (1) a defined endpoint, (2) a defined purpose, (3) a description of the underlying rationale, (4) a description of the individual information sources used, (5) a description of how data from the individual information sources are processed, (6) a consideration of the known uncertainties (and in each case, a description of the magnitude of each source of uncertainty).

AOP-Supported IATA Case Study: Skin Sensitization

The AOP for skin sensitization has been well-described, and several assays have been identified that can query the MIE and upstream KEs, and there is quite a bit of evidence substantiating the prediction of the AO by measuring various combinations of these KEs (OECD 2012a, b). There are also a number of different IATA that have been developed to assess skin sensitization (e.g. Natsch et al. 2013; Ramirez et al. 2016; OECD 2016c) (Fig. 3). Nearly all sensitizers are molecules that are or can become electrophiles and will react covalently with proteins. If these substances are exposed to and can penetrate skin, they are likely to cause allergic reactions in humans. Several computer models exist that relate the structure of a molecule to its potential to become an electrophile (Quantitative Structure Activity Relationships or QSARs), and for many molecules, can accurately predict skin sensitizing potential. Several QSARs and in vitro test methods exist to look at the MIE (covalent reaction with proteins) and two early KE (dendritic cell and keratinocyte activation). IATA using combinations of one or more of these assays have been evaluated for regulatory application, some of which outperform animal tests to predict human skin sensitization (Bauch et al 2012; Natsch et al. 2013; OECD 2016c).

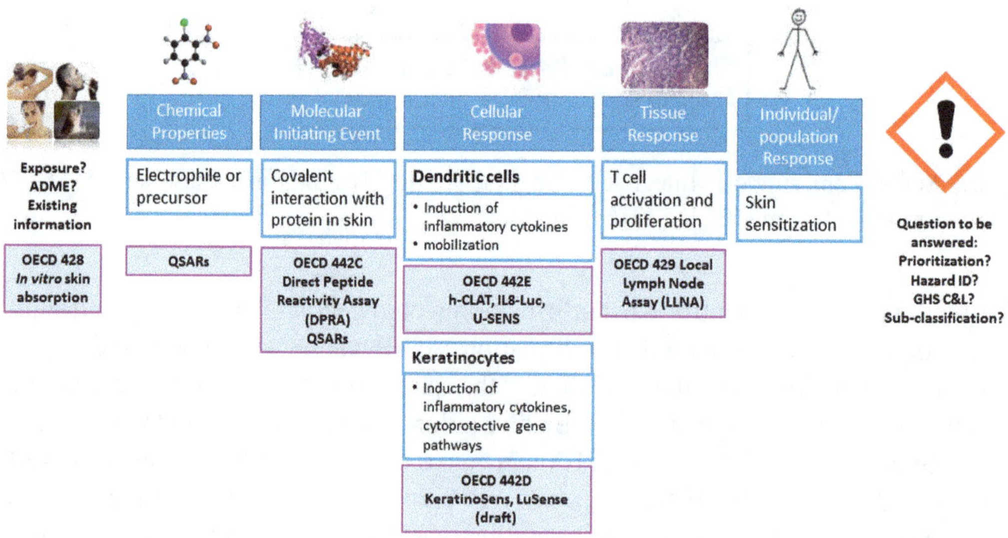

Fig. 3. Skin sensitization AOP and validated methods to assess various KEs (pink outlined boxes).

To facilitate regulatory uptake of IATA for skin sensitization, the International Cooperation on Alternative Test Methods (ICATM), in collaboration with OECD and the European Commission's Joint Research Centre, held a workshop on the International Regulatory Applicability and Acceptance of Alternative Approaches to Skin Sensitization Assessment of Chemicals (Kleinstreuer et al. 2017). Attendees, which included 40 regulators and scientists from 12 countries, concluded that in vitro methods are available that are adequate for use within an IATA to predict skin sensitization for regulatory purposes, but that a number of barriers remain to be surmounted, including: a lack of familiarity and need for training in the methods and development of clear guidance for application of multiple IATA. A recommendation was for OECD to develop a performance-based test guideline for skin sensitization IATA. To follow on this workshop, the OECD is coordinating a project, led by the US ICCVAM and Environmental Protection Agency and the EC JRC, to evaluate the 12 IATA described in OECD Guidance Document 256 (OECD 2016c). A special OECD workshop was held in Dec 2017 to review the progress and obtain input from the OECD national coordinators of the test guideline program. Results of the study are expected in mid 2018.

Summary

AOPs can support decision making, including for regulatory application, and in several ways. AOPs can: support WoE evaluations; form the basis for integrated approaches to testing and assessment; provide the basis for biological hypothesis to identify what information would be most helpful for decreasing uncertainty in a given situation; provide transparent communication of the information and uncertainty that underlie decisions; form the basis for development of predictive models. The OECD is coordinating an AOP KB for collecting and assessing information related to AOPs. The AOP Wiki is a crowd-sourcing platform that is open to all interested parties and guidance materials and training courses to assist in use are freely available. Participation in the wiki should be promoted as the more expert input into the wiki, the more useful the knowledgebase will become. IATA are designed to streamline regulatory decision making. OECD has created a number of guidance documents to assist with the development and review of IATA. Development of IATA begin with problem formulation that includes consideration of the regulatory context and gathering of all existing relevant information. IATA are hypothesis-driven and can be supported by AOPs. There can be more than one IATA to answer a given question, and that necessitates the development of specific cases of IATA, or defined approaches, that consist of defined methods and data interpretation procedures, for regulatory application. OECD and member organizations are developing case studies of defined approaches, beginning with skin sensitization.

References

Bauch C, Kolle SN, Ramirez T, Eltze T, Fabian E, Mehling A, Teubner W, van Ravenzwaay B, Landsiedel R (2012) Putting the parts together: combining in vitro methods to test for skin sensitizing potentials. Regul Toxicol Pharmacol 63(3):489–504. https://doi.org/10.1016/j.yrtph.2012.05.013. (Erratum in: Regul Toxicol Pharmacol 64(2):285 2012)

Kleinstreuer N, Strickland J, Casati S, Barroso J, Zuang V, Lowit A, Matheson J, Allen D, Casey W, Whelan M (2017) Evaluating defined approaches to testing and assessment of skin sensitization potential. Presented at the society of toxicology annual meeting, March 12–16, Baltimore, MD. https://ntp.niehs.nih.gov/iccvam/meetings/sot17/kleinstreuer-sotposter1-fd.pdf. Acccssed 31 Jan 2018

Meek ME, Palermo CM, Bachman AN, North CM, Lewis RJ (2014) Mode of action human relevance (MOA/HR) framework—evolution of the bradford hill considerations and comparative analysis of weight of evidence. Toxicol, Appl. https://doi.org/10.1002/jat.2984

National Research Council (2007) Toxicity testing in the 21st century: a vision and a strategy. National Academy of Sciences, Washington, DC, USA

Natsch A, Ryan CA, Foertsch L, Emter R, Jaworska J, Gerberick F, Kern P (2013) A dataset on 145 chemicals tested in alternative assays for skin sensitization undergoing prevalidation. J Appl Toxicol 33:1337–1352. https://doi.org/10.1002/jat.2868

OECD (2012a) The adverse outcome pathway for skin sensitisation initiated by covalent binding to proteins, part 1: scientific evidence. Series on Testing and Assessment, No. 168. OECD, Paris, France

OECD (2012b) The adverse outcome pathway for skin sensitisation initiated by covalent binding to proteins, part 2: use of the AOP to develop chemical categories and integrated assessment and testing. Series on Testing and Assessment, No. 168. OECD, Paris, France

OECD (2018) Users' Handbook supplement to the guidance document for developing and assessing adverse outcome pathways. OECD Series on Adverse Outcome Pathways, No. 1, OECD Publishing, Paris. http://dx.doi.org/10.1787/5jlv1m9d1g32-en

OECD (2016a) Reporting of defined approaches to be used within integrated approaches to testing and assessment. Series on Testing and Assessment, No. 255. OECD Publishing, Paris

OECD (2016b) Use of adverse outcome pathways in developing integrated approaches to testing and assessment (IATA). Series on Testing and Assessment, No. 260. OECD Publishing, Paris

OECD (2016c) Guidance document on the reporting of defined approaches and individual information sources to be used within integrated approaches to testing and assessment (IATA) for skin sensitisation. Series on Testing and Assessment, No. 256. OECD Publishing, Paris

Ramirez T, Stein N, Aumann A, Remus T, Edwards A, Norman KG, Ryan C, Bader JE, Fehr M, Burleson F, Foertsch L, Wang X, Gerberick F, Beilstein P, Hoffmann S, Mehling A, van Ravenzwaay B, Landsiedel R (2016) Intra- and inter-laboratory reproducibility and accuracy of the LuSens assay: a reporter gene-cell line to detect keratinocyte activation by skin sensitizers. Toxicol Vitr 32:278–286

Sachana M, Leinala E (2017) Approaching chemical safety assessment through application of integrated approaches to testing and assessment: combining mechanistic information derived from adverse outcome pathways and alternative methods. Appl Vitr Toxicol 3(3): 227–233

Villeneuve DL, Crump D, Garcia-Reyero N, Hecker M, Hutchinson TH, LaLone CA, Landesmann B, Lettieri T, Munn S, Nepelska M, Ottinger MA, Vergauwen L, M Whelan (2014) Adverse outcome pathway (AOP) development I: strategies and principles. Toxicol Sci 142:312–320

Mechanism-Based Evaluation System for Hepato- and Nephrotoxicity or Carcinogenicity Using Omics Technology

Fumiyo Saito(✉)

Chemicals Assessment and Research Center, Chemicals Evaluation and Research Institute (CERI), Saitama, Japan
saito-fumiyo@ceri.jp

Abstract. We have been developing a carcinogenicity prediction system based on gene expression profiles focusing on omics technology to enable mechanism-based evaluations of toxicity to reduce the numbers of animals and toxicological endpoints required by animal studies. Here, we report the development of a mechanism-based evaluation system focused on chemically induced hepato- and nephrotoxicity or hepatic and renal carcinogenicity using a gene expression analysis with a DNA microarray. As a case study, the mode-of-action (MoA)/adverse outcome pathway (AOP) was constructed from the gene expression profiles and histopathological findings of carbon tetrachloride and cisplatin for hepatotoxicity and nephrotoxicity, respectively. Consequently, we developed an advanced toxicity evaluation system for hepato- and nephrotoxicity or hepatic and renal carcinogenicity based on the toxicity mechanisms. We also developed a new prediction system named "CARCINOscreen®" for evaluating the carcinogenic potentials of chemicals using the gene expression profiles of liver and kidney tissues from rats after a 28-day repeated administration. The prediction system could predict the carcinogenicity potential of a training chemical set including carcinogens and non-carcinogens with an accuracy of more than 90%. The marker genes established in this study are promising for the development of new effective in vitro testing methods in the future.

Keywords: Adverse outcome pathway (AOP) · Gene expression profiles · Hepatotoxicity · Nephrotoxicity · Carcinogenicity CARCINOscreen®

Introduction

Of the more than 80,000 chemicals in commerce, rigorous safety testing and risk assessment has been carried on relatively few. As an example, rodent carcinogenicity test data available for less than 1,000 compounds in the US National Toxicology Program database. The carcinogenicity of chemicals in our environment is an important health hazard to humans. Carcinogenicity studies using rodents have long been the standard for evaluating the carcinogenic potential of chemicals [1]; however, such studies are time-consuming, expensive, and require large numbers of experimental animals. Therefore, the carcinogenic potential of many important chemicals remains

H. Kojima et al. (Eds.): *Alternatives to Animal Testing*, pp. 91–104, 2019.
https://doi.org/10.1007/978-981-13-2447-5_12

untested. In addition to the carcinogenic potential, the hepatotoxicity and nephrotoxicity of xenobiotics, which include classical drugs, herbal medicines, and chemical products, represents a significant cause of liver and kidney diseases [2, 3]. To evaluate hazards of a compound, various toxicity studies are needed, leading to problems such as a high cost and long test period in regulatory sciences. The test guideline known as the "repeated dose 28-day oral toxicity study in rodents" (TG 407) adopted by the Organization for Economic Co-operation and Development (OECD) is used mainly in Japan and Europe as a screening toxicity test. If an initial response, such as a change in a gene expression level associated with toxic effects, could be detected, a single animal study might be capable of predicting various toxicity endpoints, including long-term toxicity. Under these circumstances, the development of an efficient hazard assessment system for chemicals is needed. Moreover, the promotion of a "3Rs" policy and the development of promising in vitro alternative test methods, are both progressing in toxicological studies.

Omics technology, such as gene expression analyses, can be used effectively for the identification and prediction of hazards. Toxicogenomics has been established as a powerful tool for elucidating the mechanisms of chemical toxicity, such as carcinogenicity [4–6], hepatotoxicity [7, 8] and nephrotoxicity [9, 10]. However, numerous unknown pathways or gene networks that lead to toxicity exist. For a better understanding of adverse outcome pathways (AOPs) and the expansion of mode of action (MoA) applications, the elucidation of pathways/networks or biomarkers to detect or predict *in vivo* toxicity is needed.

We participated in a 5-year ARCH-Tox project conducted by the Ministry of Economy, Trade and Industry (METI) in Japan with the aim of developing a new testing approach that would enable the evaluation of multiple endpoints (hepatotoxicity/nephrotoxicity, carcinogenicity and neurotoxicity) in a single 28-day repeated dose toxicity study using sets of marker genes selected based on toxicity mechanism such as MoAs or AOPs. Mechanism-based analysis using omics technology is expected to reveal new MoAs or AOPs, leading to the development of new *in vitro* assays.

Chemicals, Animal Test and Microarray Analysis

A total of 100 chemicals, consisting of 68 chemicals used in prediction systems examining hepatic carcinogenicity and 32 chemicals commonly used in prediction systems examining renal carcinogenicity and detection systems for hepatotoxicity and nephrotoxicity, were selected from among chemicals used in previous studies [11–13]. The number of test compounds used in each experiment is shown in Fig. 1a.

Four-week-old specific-pathogen-free (SPF) male Crl:CD (SD) rats and Fischer 344 (F344) rats were obtained from Charles River Laboratories Japan, Inc. (Kanagawa, Japan). The rats were treated with the test compounds in a suitable vehicle by gavage for 28 days. The animals were then sacrificed by exsanguination under anesthesia with CO_2–O_2 (4:1) or isoflurane gas inhalation 24 h after the final administration, and the livers were immediately excised and weighed. Then, the left lateral lobe of the liver was sliced and immediately placed in RNA*later*® (Ambion, Austin, TX, USA) for RNA extraction; the remaining liver sample was submitted for histopathological examination. All the animals were treated in compliance with the applicable animal

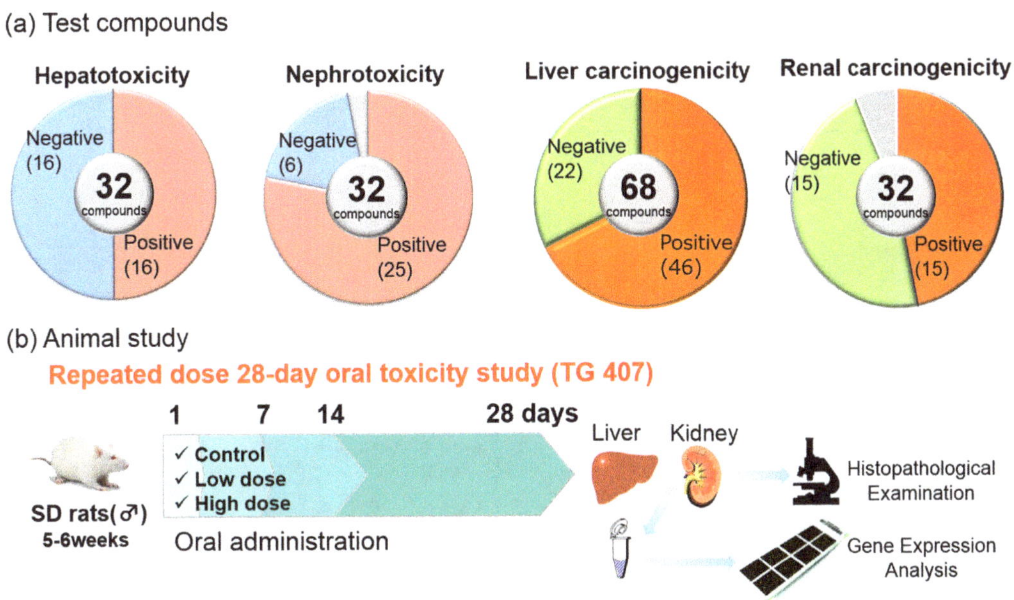

Fig. 1. Number of test compounds used in each experiment and animal study design **a** Test compounds: Sixty-eight chemicals were used to develop a prediction system for hepatic carcinogenicity, and 32 chemicals were used to develop prediction systems for renal carcinogenicity and detection systems for hepatotoxicity and nephrotoxicity. **b** Animal study: The gene expression profiles of liver and kidney tissues were detected after a 28-day repeated dose toxicity study in male Crl:CD (SD) rats

Table 1. Histopathological findings of liver (CCl_4)

Findings	Grade	0 mg/kg/day				20 mg/kg/day				100 mg/kg/day			
		D1	D7	D14	D28	D1	D7	D14	D28	D1	D7	D14	D28
Fatty degeneration, /Hepatocyte/ Centrilobular	—	4	4	4	5	3	0	0	0	0	0	0	0
	±	0	0	0	0	1	1	0	0	4	0	0	0
	+	0	0	0	0	0	1	4	5	0	1	2	2
	++	0	0	0	0	0	2	0	0	0	3	2	2
	+++	0	0	0	0	0	0	0	0	0	0	0	1
Hydropic degeneration, Hepatocyte/ Centrilobular	—	4	4	4	5	4	4	4	5	3	1	0	0
	±	0	0	0	0	0	0	0	0	1	0	0	0
	+	0	0	0	0	0	0	0	0	0	3	3	3
	++	0	0	0	0	0	0	0	0	0	0	1	2
Microgranuloma	—	4	4	4	5	4	0	0	0	4	0	0	1
	+	0	0	0	0	0	1	2	5	0	4	2	0
	++	0	0	0	0	0	3	2	0	0	0	2	4
Mitosis, increased	—	4	4	4	5	4	4	2	3	4	2	0	1
	+	0	0	0	0	0	0	1	2	0	0	3	1
	++	0	0	0	0	0	0	1	0	0	2	1	3
Single cell necrosis, Hepatocyte/ Centrilobular	—	4	4	4	5	4	4	4	5	1	4	4	5
	+	0	0	0	0	0	0	0	0	3	0	0	0

-: no remarkable, ±:mild, +: slight, ++: moderate, +++: marked.

Numbers indicate the number of animals whose histopathological findings of liver were observed in each treatment group (4 animals on days 1, 7, and 14, and 5 animals on days 28).

welfare regulations (Declaration of Helsinki [2000] and guidelines for animal experiments at CERI according to LABORATORY ANIMAL SCIENCE [1987] published by the American Association for Laboratory Animal Science). The experimental design and the results of histopathological findings is shown in Fig. 1b and Tables 1 and 2, respectively.

Table 2. Histopathological findings of kidney (cisplatin)

Findings	Grade	0 mg/kg/day				0.15 mg/kg/day				0.75 mg/kg/day			
		D1	D7	D14	D28	D1	D7	D14	D28	D1	D7	D14	D28
Single cell necrosis / Renal tube/ Cortico-medullary junction	—	4	4	4	5	4	4	4	5	4	3	2	1
	+	0	0	0	0	0	0	0	0	0	1	3	2
	++	0	0	0	0	0	0	0	0	0	0	0	2
Single cell necrosis / Renal tube/ Inner medullar	—	4	4	4	5	4	4	4	5	4	4	4	2
	+	0	0	0	0	0	0	0	0	0	0	0	2
	++	0	0	0	0	0	0	0	0	0	0	0	1
Degeneration / Renal tube/ Cortex, Cortico-medullary junction	—	4	4	4	5	4	4	4	5	4	3	1	5
	+	0	0	0	0	0	0	0	0	0	1	3	0
	++	0	0	0	0	0	0	0	0	0	0	0	0
Karyomegaly / Renal tube/ Cortico-medullary junction	—	4	4	4	5	4	4	4	5	4	4	4	0
	+	0	0	0	0	0	0	0	0	0	0	0	0
	++	0	0	0	0	0	0	0	0	0	0	0	5
Karyomegaly / Renal tube/ Inner medullar	—	4	4	4	5	4	4	4	5	4	4	4	2
	+	0	0	0	0	0	0	0	0	0	0	0	3
	++	0	0	0	0	0	0	0	0	0	0	0	0
Dilation / Renal pelvis	—	4	4	4	5	4	4	4	5	4	3	3	5
	+	0	0	0	0	0	0	0	0	0	0	1	0
	++	0	0	0	0	0	0	0	0	0	1	0	0
Dilation / Renal tube/ Cortico-medullary junction	—	4	4	4	5	4	4	4	5	4	4	4	0
	+	0	0	0	0	0	0	0	0	0	0	0	1
	++	0	0	0	0	0	0	0	0	0	0	0	2
	+++	0	0	0	0	0	0	0	0	0	0	0	2
Regeneration / Renal tube/ Cortico-medullary junction	—	4	4	4	5	4	4	4	4	4	4	0	0
	+	0	0	0	0	0	0	0	1	0	0	1	0
	++	0	0	0	0	0	0	0	0	0	0	3	0
	++	0	0	0	0	0	0	0	0	0	0	0	5
Regeneration / Renal tube/Inner medullar	—	4	4	4	5	4	4	4	5	4	4	4	0
	+	0	0	0	0	0	0	0	0	0	0	0	3
	++	0	0	0	0	0	0	0	0	0	0	0	2

-: no remarkable, +: slight, ++: moderate, +++: marked.
Numbers indicate the number of animals whose histopathological findings of kidney were observed in each treatment group (4 animals on days 1, 7, and 14, and 5 animals on days 28).

Total RNA was extracted from the liver samples using QIAzol (Qiagen, Hilden, Germany) and the RNeasy Mini Kit or miRNeasy Mini Kit (Qiagen), in accordance with the manufacturer's protocol. The quality of the RNA samples was examined using the Agilent 2100 Bioanalyzer (Agilent Technologies, Santa Clara, CA, USA), and undegraded RNA samples were used for the experiments; for this study, we used RNA samples with RIN values of > 7.0 as an index of the high purity and integrity of the RNA samples.

Microarray analysis was performed as described previously [12]. Briefly, three types of custom arrays, Toxarray III ver.2 and Agilent Whole Rat Genome Microarrays 8 × 60 K Toxplus ver.1 and ver.2, and the gene-expression-based carcinogenicity prediction system CARCINOscreen® were used for the microarray analysis. Global normalization was applied to one-color microarray data using GeneSpring GX 10 (Agilent Technologies). Lowess normalization was applied to two-color microarray data using Feature Extraction Software 9.5.3.1 (Agilent Technologies). The signal $\log_2$ ratio of the administration group vs. the vehicle control group was calculated using the mean normalized signal intensity in each group. The pathway or functional analysis for the DNA microarray data was performed using Ingenuity Pathways Analysis (IPA) software (Qiagen).

AOP-Based Mechanism of Hepatotoxicity Suggested by Case Study with Carbon Tetrachloride

The liver has long been considered the major target organ for most of the chemicals implicated in eliciting toxic effects following environmental exposure. Hepatotoxicity represents a major regulatory issue, and the pathophysiologic mechanisms of hepatotoxicity are still being explored and include both hepatocellular and extracellular mechanisms. We investigated the mechanism of hepatotoxicity induced by carbon tetrachloride (CCl_4), which is a well-known hepatotoxin. CCl_4 reportedly damages liver cell mitochondria and causes the failed transport of fatty acids as phospholipids [14]. We attempted to create an AOP for liver fibrosis induced by CCl_4 using gene expression data and histopathological data obtained in our studies as well as previously reported information [14]. A previous study reported that CCl_4 was biotransformed by the cytochrome P450 system in the endoplasmic reticulum to produce trichloromethyl free radical ($CCl^{\cdot}_3$) [15]. This $CCl^{\cdot}_3$ then combined with cellular lipids and proteins to form trichloromethyl peroxyl free radical, which attacks lipids on the membrane of the endoplasmic reticulum as a molecular initiating event (MIE). Thus, trichloromethyl peroxyl free radical is thought to lead to lipid peroxidation [15]. In the results of our case study using CCl_4., Cyp2c12 and Cyp4f5 were upregulated and cholesterol biosynthesis appeared to be activated, while fatty acid β-oxidation appeared to be downregulated in association with a 1-day treatment with CCl_4. A functional analysis using IPA software of significantly downregulated genes in the liver after the administration of CCl_4 showed that these genes were strongly correlated with fatty acid metabolism, transport of lipid and cleavage of lipid became with the severity depending on the administration period (Fig. 2). After 7 days of administration or thereafter, the significantly upregulated genes were strongly correlated with increases in the synthesis of DNA, DNA replication and chromosomal congression as well as the p63 signaling pathway and the G2/M DNA damage checkpoint pathway (data not shown). Histopathologically, fatty degeneration and centrilobular hydropic degeneration were observed by macroscopic examination on the first day of administration. Furthermore,

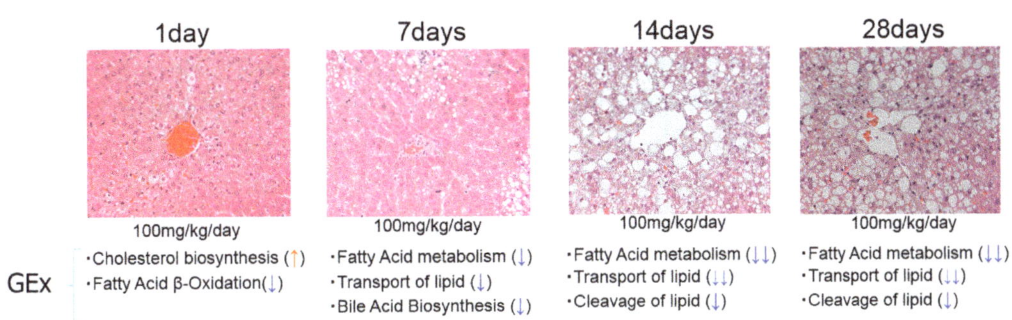

Fig. 2. Histopathological changes and functional analysis of DNA microarray data obtained after the oral administration of carbon tetrachloride (CCl4). The *red* and *blue* arrows indicate a significant functional analysis using IPA software for the up- and downregulated genes, respectively. The number of arrows shows the degree of relevance of these function and gene expression changes

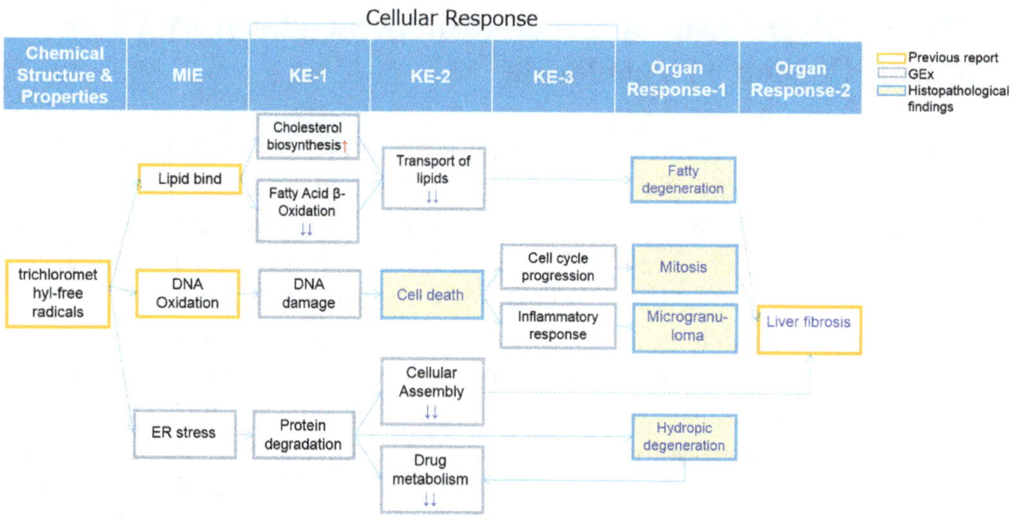

Fig. 3. AOP-based mechanisms of hepatotoxicity of carbon tetrachloride (CCl4). MIE: molecular initiating event, KE: key event, GEx: Gene expression data. The *red* and *blue* arrows indicate the significance of a functional analysis using IPA software for the up- and downregulated genes, respectively. The number of arrows shows the degree of relevance of these function and gene expression changes

microgranuloma, mitosis and single cell necrosis in the centrilobular area were observed, and the degree of severity increased with the dose and administration period (Table 1). We constructed AOP-based hepatotoxicity mechanisms of CCl_4 using these multifaceted considerations, and the mechanism map is shown in Fig. 3.

AOP-Based Mechanism of Nephrotoxicity Suggested by Case Study with Cisplatin

Recent studies have demonstrated that the kidney is also an important target of injury after chemical exposure, although substantial gaps in knowledge remain regarding the effects of environmental chemicals on specific aspects of kidney function [16, 17]. Cisplatin is a potent anticancer drug that is widely used in chemotherapy. However, adverse effects in normal tissues and organs, notably nephrotoxicity in the kidneys, limit the use of cisplatin and related platinum-based therapeutics. Recent research has shed significant new light on the mechanism of cisplatin nephrotoxicity, especially on the signaling pathways leading to tubular cell death and inflammation [18]. As a case study of nephrotoxicity, we administered cisplatin to male rats for 28 days; kidney samples were then obtained and anatomically separated into the papilla, inner medulla, outer medulla, and cortex, which have different structures and functions, and gene expression analyses were performed for each of these renal anatomic regions, since the marked morphological, functional and biochemical heterogeneity of the kidney accounts for the site-specific toxicity of several drugs and xenobiotics [19]. In our previous DNA microarray study, no significant variations for each renal anatomic region were seen between the left and right kidneys or among individuals (data not shown). Nevertheless, the gene expression profiles differed in each renal anatomic region, and the DNA microarray data of the outer medulla and cortex were used to analyze the nephrotoxicity of cisplatin. The major focus in renal damage research is on proximal tubule toxicity, where the majority of the reabsorption of drug metabolites occurs, and the proximal tubules of the nephron in animals including the proximal convoluted tubules, which are situated in the cortical labyrinth and are connected directly to the proximal straight tubules in the inner cortex and outer stripe of the outer medulla [19]. Cisplatin has been suggested to produce reactive oxygen species (ROS) via NADPH oxidase activation [20]. ROS are highly reactive molecules that can damage cell structures such as carbohydrates, nucleic acids, lipids, and proteins and alter their functions [21]. In this gene expression data, Nrf2, Gpx2, Ho-1, Scarb1, Gstm3, and Mgst2, which are concerned with the NRF2-mediated oxidative stress response, were significantly upregulated, supporting the MIE of cisplatin, *i.e.* the oxidation of DNA, proteins, lipids, and co-factors (data not shown). A functional analysis using IPA software of significantly upregulated genes in the outer medulla of the kidney after the administration of cisplatin showed that these genes were strongly correlated with cell death and survival, inflammatory disease, cellular growth and proliferation, organismal injury and abnormalities, and apoptosis (data not shown). The downregulated genes were involved in amino acid metabolism, lipid metabolism, vitamin and mineral metabolism, drug metabolism, and molecular transport, which is involved in basic renal function (data not shown). In particular, many genes expressed in the outer medulla and cortex related to oxidative phosphorylation, were downregulated, resulting in mitochondrial dysfunction (Fig. 4). The proximal tubule of the kidney has three morphologically distinct segments, S_1, S_2, and S_3, which can be distinguished as the pars convoluta and the pars recta of the proximal tubule [22]. Epithelial cells in the S_1 segments possess a tall brush border, a well-developed vacuolar lysosomal system, and many long mitochondria that fill the basal portion of the cell. The S_2 segments are not as tall as the S_1 segments. The S_3 cells have rare apical vacuoles and fewer and smaller mitochondria than the S_1 and S_2 cells [22]. These observations suggest that the administration of cisplatin leads to kidney injury and abnormalities. Histopathologically, after 7 days of administration or longer, single cell necrosis of the proximal tubule in the cortico-medullary junction or the inner medulla was observed microscopically. Furthermore, degeneration, karyomegaly, dilation, and regeneration were observed, and the degree of severity increased with the dose and administration period (Table 2). We constructed an AOP-based hepatotoxicity mechanism for cisplatin using these multifaceted considerations, as shown in Fig. 5.

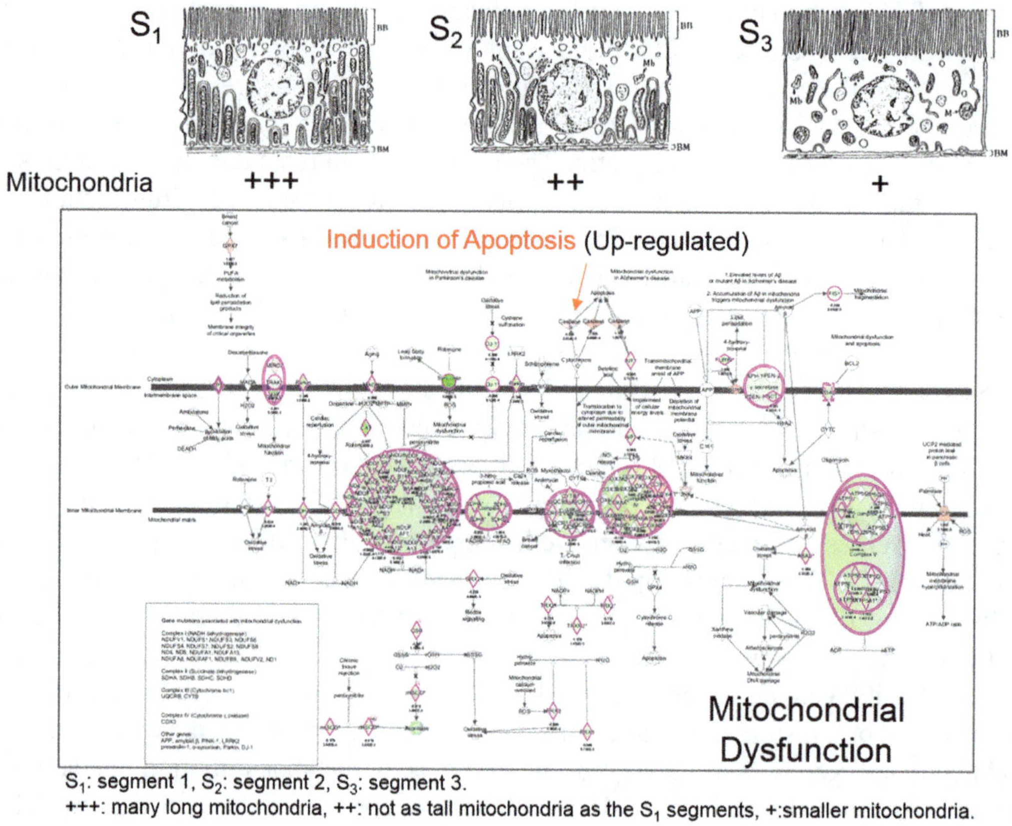

Fig. 4. An example of a pathway analysis of DNA microarray data obtained after the intraperitoneal administration of cisplatin. The *red* and *green* colored objects indicate the up- and downregulated genes, respectively

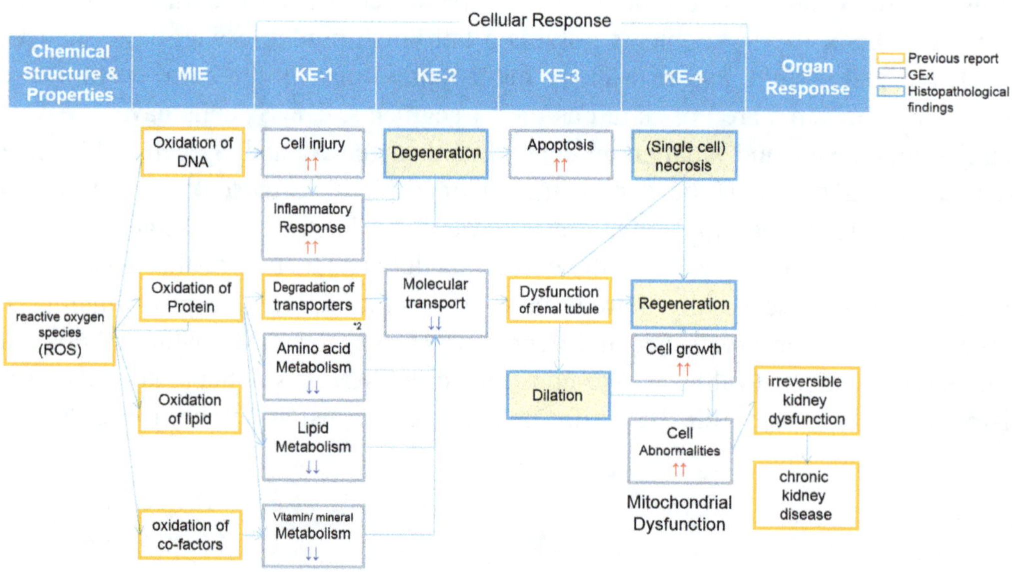

Fig. 5. AOP-based mechanisms of nephrotoxicity of cisplatin. MIE: molecular initiating event, KE: key event. The *red* and *blue* arrows indicate the significance of a functional analysis using IPA software for the up- and downregulated genes, respectively. The number of arrows shows the degree of relevance of these function and gene expression changes

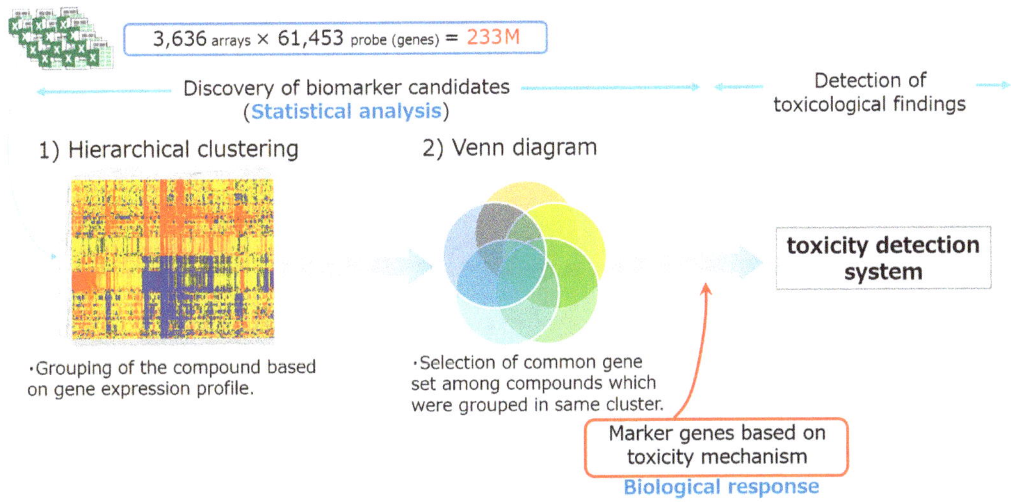

Fig. 6. Strategy of a detection system for hepato- and nephrotoxicity. To discover biomarker candidates, microarray data was analyzed using hierarchical clustering to group compounds based on gene expression profiles, and common gene sets among the compounds that were grouped in the same cluster were selected and used in a Venn diagram. Furthermore, marker genes based on toxicity mechanisms were selected based on the results of an AOP-based mechanisms analysis of hepato- and nephrotoxicity, and toxicity detection systems were constructed for each toxicological finding

Table 3. Toxicological findings and number of detection genes for hepato- and nephrotoxicity

Organ	Toxicological findings		Detection genes
Liver	Centrilobular	Fatty degeneration	8
	Periportal		36
	–	Cell death	14
	Centrilobular	Hypertrophy	24
	Diffuse		18
Kidney	Proximal tubule	Vacuolization	3
	Proximal tubule	Anisonucleosis	4
	Proximal tubule	Pyknosis	4
	Proximal tubule	Cell death	10
	Papilla	necrosis	9

Detection System for Hepato- and Nephrotoxicity

We attempted to develop a detection system for hepato- and nephrotoxicity using DNA microarray data; the strategy used to construct the detection system is shown in Fig. 6. We focused on frequently listed toxicity findings in the Hazard Evaluation Support System Integrated Platform database (HESS-DB: http://www.nite.go.jp/en/chem/qsar/hess-e.html), which contains information on toxicity and metabolism released in Japan. We then chose five toxicological findings for each toxicity: centrilobular fatty

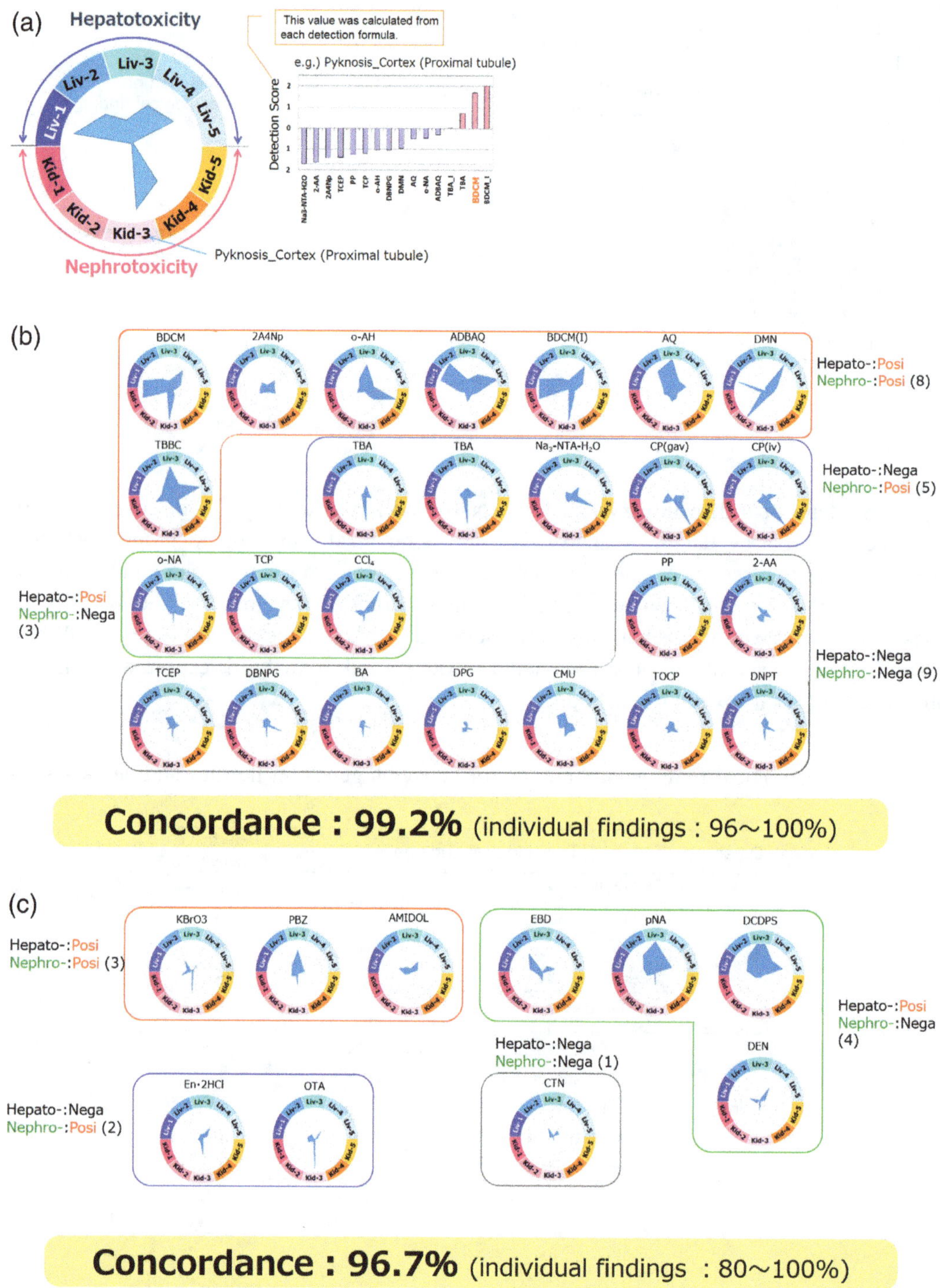

Fig. 7. Detection results for hepato- and nephrotoxicity. **a** Radar chart model of the detection system: The detection score was calculated using a support vector machine with the detection genes. Each detection score for the five toxicological findings in the liver and kidney was plotted in the upper and lower areas of the radar chart, respectively. **b** Results of training data (25 tests/22 compounds), **c** Results of validation data (10 tests/10 compounds): Liv-1: centrilobular fatty degeneration, Liv-2: periportal fatty degeneration, Liv-3: cell death, Liv-4: centrilobular hypertrophy, Liv-5: hypertrophy (diffuse). Kid-1: vacuolization of proximal tubule, Kid-2: anisonucleosis of proximal tubule, Kid-3: pyknosis of proximal tubule, Kid-4: cell death of proximal tubule, Kid-5: necrosis of papilla

degeneration, periportal fatty degeneration, cell death, centrilobular hypertrophy, and hypertrophy (diffuse) for hepatotoxicity, and vacuolization of the proximal tubule, anisonucleosis of the proximal tubule, pyknosis of the proximal tubule, cell death of the proximal tubule, and necrosis of the papilla for nephrotoxicity. The detection formula was generated using a support vector machine with detection genes selected from 22 training chemicals (25 tests) datasets, and a predictive score was then calculated to detect the hepato- or nephrotoxicity potentials of the tested chemicals. The detection genes were selected for each toxicological finding: 8–36 genes for hepatotoxicity and 3–10 genes for nephrotoxicity (Table 3). The potential score for each toxicological finding was shown in a radar chart model that allowed the visualization of multiple toxicity findings at a glance (Fig. 7a). In the training data, the potential score for each toxicological finding was 96%–100%, resulting in a 99.2% total concordance (Fig. 7b). In the validation data for ten chemicals, the potential score for each toxicological finding was 80%–100%, resulting in a 96.7% total concordance (Fig. 7c).

Prediction System for Hepatic and Renal Carcinogenicity: CARCINOscreen®

Carcinogenicity is one of the most serious toxic effects of chemicals, and highly accurate methods for predicting carcinogens are strongly desired for the assessment on human health. We previously developed a prediction system named "CARCINOscreen®" for evaluating the carcinogenic potentials of chemicals using the gene expression profiles of liver tissues from rats after a 28-day repeated dose toxicity study [12]. The prediction formula was generated using a support vector machine with predictive genes selected from 68 training chemical datasets; a predictive score was then calculated to predict the carcinogenic potentials of the tested chemicals. To ensure the accuracy of the prediction system, the chemicals were divided into three groups (Groups 1 to 3) according to the resulting hepatic gene expression profiles, and a prediction formula was generated for each group. The prediction system was capable of predicting the carcinogenicity of the training carcinogens and the non-carcinogens with an accuracy of 92.9%–100%. The final prediction result was determined based on the maximum prediction value obtained with three independent prediction formulas to establish the CARCINOscreen®. The system was able to accurately predict carcinogenicity in rats in 94.1% of the 68 training chemicals [12]. Furthermore, we attempted to develop a quantitative PCR (qPCR)-based system as an alternative to the microarray-based CARCINOscreen® [23]. The prediction accuracies of the qPCR-based alternative for training- and validation-phase trials were 82.8% and 86.4%, respectively [23].

Recently, we reported a renal carcinogenicity prediction system to predict chemical carcinogenicity in rats; a 28-day repeated-dose test was performed using male Crl:CD (SD) rats with 12 carcinogens and 10 non-carcinogens as the training dataset and five carcinogens and five non-carcinogens as the validation dataset [13]. In this prediction system, the prediction accuracies for the training and the validation datasets were calculated to be 100% and 90%, respectively, while 4-hydroxy-*m*-phenylenediammonium dichloride (AMIDOL), a known non-renal carcinogen, was judged as being positive. Among the predictive genes, Hamp and Ranbp1 are known to be important for cell growth and cell cycle regulation, which are important events in carcinogenesis. Given our current limited knowledge of the genes responsible for renal carcinogenesis, the identification of candidate genes for chemical-induced renal carcinogenicity using this gene expression-based prediction method represents a promising advance in renal carcinogen identification [13].

Concluding Remarks

In hepatotoxicity and nephrotoxicity, marker genes can be selected based on toxicity mechanisms such as MoA or AOP, enabling a detection accuracy of more than 90% for five kinds of toxicity findings in both the liver and kidney. For carcinogenicity, the CARCINOscreen® system predicted the carcinogenic potential of a training compound set that included non-carcinogens with a more than 90% accuracy for the liver and kidney. Furthermore, we developed a qPCR-based prediction system as an alternative to the microarray-based CARCINOscreen® for rat liver carcinogenicity. The prediction performance of the qPCR-based CARCINOscreen®, as well as its user-friendliness and cost effectiveness, suggests that this method is promising for application in primary health hazard assessments. These results suggested that omics technology, such as gene expression analysis, can be used effectively for hazard identification and prediction. From now on, the application of urine and blood samples, which are non- or semi-invasive to animals, might be more important as a contribution to the 3Rs policy. Blood and urine samples are used in metabolomics and proteomics approaches with a high frequency, and these techniques may also be powerful tools for the identification of toxicity mechanisms and to resolve issues in which changes in gene expression levels are not always correlated with the phenotypes.

Acknowledgement. This study was supported by a grant from the Ministry of Economy, Trade and Industry, Japan (ARCH-Tox).

References

1. Chhabra RS, Huff JE, Schwetz BS, Selkirk J (1990) An overview of prechronic and chronic toxicity/carcinogenicity experimental study designs and criteria used by the National Toxicology Program. Environ Health Perspect 86:313–321
2. Robert CJ, Stephen MR (2015) Hepatotoxicity: toxic effects on the liver. In: Robert CJ, Stephen MR, Lawrence HL (eds) Principles of toxicology: environmental and industrial applications, 3rd edn. Wiley, New York, pp 125–138
3. Lawrence HL (2015) Nephrotoxicity: toxic responses of the kidney. In: Robert CJ, Stephen MR, Lawrence HL (eds) Principles of toxicology: environmental and industrial applications, 3rd edn. Wiley, New York, pp 139–155
4. Ellinger-Ziegelbauer H, Gmuender H, Bandenburg A, Ahr HJ (2008) Prediction of a carcinogenic potential of rat hepatocarcinogen using toxicogenomics analysis of short-term in vivo studies. Mutat Res 637(1–2):23–39

5. Fielden MR, Adai A, Dunn RT 2nd, Olaharski A, Searfoss G, Sina J, Aubrecht J, Boitier E, Nioi P, Auerbach S, Jacobson-Kram D, Raghavan N, Yang Y, Kincaid A, Sherlock J, Chen SJ, Car B, Predictive Safety Testing Consortium, Carcinogenicity Working Group (2011) Development and evaluation of a genomic signature for the prediction and mechanistic assessment of nongenotoxic hepatocarcinogens in the rat. Toxicol Sci 124(1):54–74
6. Yudate HT, Kai T, Aoki M, Minowa Y, Yamada T, Kimura T, Ono A, Yamada H, Ohno Y, Urushidani T (2012) Identification of a novel set of biomarkers for evaluating phospholipidosis-inducing potential of compounds using rat liver microarray data measured 24-h after single dose administration. Toxicology 295(1–3):1–7
7. Singh P, Mishra SK, Noel S, Sharma S, Rath SK (2012) Acute exposure of apigenin induces hepatotoxicity in Swiss mice. PLoS ONE 7(2):e31964
8. Sahini N, Selvaraj S, Borlak J (2014) Whole genome transcript profiling of drug induced steatosis in rats reveals a gene signature predictive of outcome. PLoS ONE 9(12):e114085
9. Marin-Kuan M, Nestler S, Verguet C, Bezençon C, Piguet D, Mansourian R, Holzwarth J, Grigorov M, Delatour T, Mantle P, Cavin C, Schilter B (2006) A toxicogenomics approach to identify new plausible epigenetic mechanisms of ochratoxin a carcinogenicity in rat. Toxicol Sci 89:20–34
10. Cui Y, Huang Q, Auman JT, Knight B, Jin X, Blanchard KT, Chou J, Jayadev S, Paules RS (2011) Genomic-derived markers for early detection of calcineurin inhibitor immunosuppressant-mediated nephrotoxicity. Toxicol Sci 124:23–34
11. Matsumoto H, Yakabe Y, Saito K, Sumida K, Sekijima M, Nakayama K, Miyaura H, Saito F, Otsuka M, Shirai T (2009) Discrimination of carcinogens by hepatic transcript profiling in rats following 28-day administration. Cancer Inform 13:253–269
12. Matsumoto H, Saito F, Takeyoshi M (2014) CARCINOscreen®: new short-term prediction method for hepatocarcinogenicity of chemicals based on hepatic transcript profiling in rats. J Toxicol Sci 39:725–734
13. Matsumoto H, Saito F, Takeyoshi M (2017) Investigation of the early-response genes in chemical-induced renal carcinogenicity for the prediction of chemical carcinogenicity in rats. J Toxicol Sci 42(2):175–181
14. Recknagel RO (1967) Carbon tetrachloride hepatotoxicity. Pharmacol Rev 19(2):145–208
15. Mayuren C, Reddy VV, Priya SV, Devi VA (2010) Protective effect of Livactine against CCl_4 and paracetamol induced hepatotoxicity in adult Wistar rats. N Am J Med Sci 2 (10):491–495
16. Bylund J, Annas A, Hellgren D, Bjurström S, Andersson H, Svanhagen A (2013) Amide hydrolysis of a novel chemical series of microsomal prostaglandin E synthase-1 inhibitors induces kidney toxicity in the rat. Drug Metab Dispos 41(3):634–641
17. Kataria A, Trasande L, Trachtman H (2015) The effects of environmental chemicals on renal function. Nat Rev Nephrol 11(10):610–625
18. Pabla N, Dong Z (2008) Cisplatin nephrotoxicity: mechanisms and renoprotective strategies. Kidney Int 73(9):994–1007
19. Hawksworth GM, McCarthy R, McGoldrick T, Stewart V, Tisocki K, Lock EA (1996) Site specific drug and xenobiotic induced renal toxicity. Arch Toxicol 18:184–192
20. Itoh T, Terazawa R, Kojima K, Nakane K, Deguchi T, Ando M, Tsukamasa Y, Ito M, Nozawa Y (2011) Cisplatin induces production of reactive oxygen species via NADPH oxidase activation in human prostate cancer cells. Free Radic Res 45(9):1033–1039

21. Birben E, Sahiner UM, Sackesen C, Erzurum S, Kalayci O (2012) Oxidative stress and antioxidant defense. World Allergy Organ J 5(1):9–19
22. Lewis BK, Brian GS (2004) Anatomy and physiological of the kidney. In: Jerry BH, Robin SG (eds) Toxicology of the kidney, 3rd edn. CRC Press, New York, pp 1–36
23. Saito F, Matsumoto H, Akahori Y, Takeyoshi M (2016) Simpler alternative to CARCINOscreen® based on quantitative PCR (qPCR). J Toxicol Sci 41(3):383–390

Alternative Methods for Developmental Toxicity Testing Using Mouse ESCs

Hee Young Kang and Eui-Bae Jeung(✉)

College of Veterinary Medicine, Chungbuk National University, 1 Chungdae-Ro, Seowon-Gu, Cheongju, Chungbuk 28644, Republic of Korea
ebjeung@chungbuk.ac.kr

Abstract. Development of an organism is accompanied by rapid and complex changes within a relatively short period, and embryotoxic chemicals administered to a mother during pregnancy can result in persistent lesions, general growth retardation, or delayed organ growth. *In vitro* toxicity tests are useful for evaluating the safety or hazards of small quantities of chemicals. Since cell death and inhibition of differentiation in mouse embryonic stem cells (ESCs) can occur within different concentration ranges of compounds, depending on the toxic potency of the compound, these cell properties can be used as guides for classifying the embryotoxicity of a compound. The use of multiple endpoints, such as assessing the inhibition of viability in ESCs ($IC_{50}ESC$) and 3T3 cells ($IC_{50}3T3$), and reduction in embryoid body (EB) area ($ID_{50}EB$), has the advantage of providing a detailed baseline for the classification of a compound's toxicity level and for establishing a prediction model that utilizes those endpoints. The EB area-based toxicity test (EBT) is an animal-free, novel drug screening system that can be useful in evaluating of various embryotoxic chemicals within a short time.

Keywords: Embryonic stem cell test · Embryoid bodies
Developmental toxicity · Prediction model

Introduction

Toxicity tests are necessary for assessing the safety or hazard levels of substances in various fields. Alternative tests based on the 3R principles (reduction, refinement, and replacement of animal use) have been proposed to overcome some of the drawbacks of animal experiments and to avoid unethical procedures [1]. Developmental toxicology is an important field in which undesirable effects on the development of an organism, including malformation, growth retardation, embryo lethality, and malfunction are assessed [2]. *In vitro* systems for testing developmental toxicity of compounds are capable of providing rapid, precise, and relevant information compared to that provided by some animal-based studies, and they are an economical approach as they are characterized by a low compound requirements and a short testing duration [3]. Embryonic stem cells (ESCs) have the capacity to self-renew and the ability to generate differentiated cells. Embryoid bodies (EBs) act at the onset of differentiation and are useful for the evaluation of developmental toxicity. The mouse embryonic stem cell test

H. Kojima et al. (Eds.): *Alternatives to Animal Testing*, pp. 105–109, 2019.
https://doi.org/10.1007/978-981-13-2447-5_13

(EST) can be used to evaluate the 50% inhibitory concentration of chemicals at three endpoints: viability of undifferentiated mouse ESCs (IC_{50}ESC), viability of mouse fibroblasts (3T3 cells; IC_{50}3T3), and differentiation of ESCs into cardiomyocytes (CMs; ID_{50}CM) (Fig. 1A green line). In our study, we used EB area to replace the assessment of cardiomyogenesis of ESCs in order to reduce the need for time-consuming and laborious processes. The replacement of CM assessment with that of EB area shortened the assessment period from 10 days to 3 days (Fig. 1A orange line). The EB area test is also referred to as the embryoid bodies test (EBT).

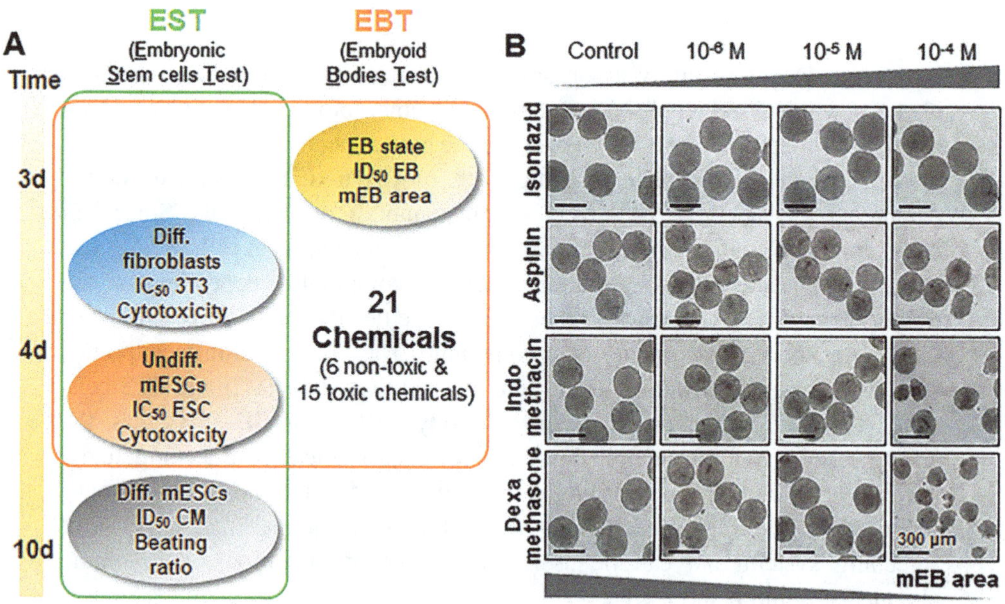

Fig. 1. Endpoints and reduction in EB area, dependent on the toxic potency of chemicals. (A) The EST evaluates the developmental toxicity of chemicals at three endpoints: Cytotoxicity in (i) ESCs. (ii) 3T3 cells, and (iii) inhibition in cardiac differentiation of ESCs at 10 days of treatment (green line). The EBT replaces cardiac differentiation endpoint with a new endpoint based on EB cross-sectional area (orange line). (B) EBs were formed over three days via the hanging drop method with 10^{-6}, 10^{-5}, or 10^{-4} M of non-toxicant (isoniazid) or toxicants (aspirin, indomethacin, or dexamethasone). Scale bars indicate 300 μm. The isoniazid-treated group maintained a EB size in 10^{-4} M treatment similar to that in the control group. Toxicant-treated groups markedly reduced the EB area at 10^{-4} M.

Materials and Methods

Twenty-one compounds (Table 1), including non-embryotoxic and embryotoxic or teratogenic chemicals, were evaluated. Cell viabilities of ESCs and 3T3 cells were measured using a cell counting kit (CCK) assay. Sectional image of EBs were photographed by a phase-contrast microscope and the EB area was analyzed by using image analysis software. The 50% inhibitory concentrations were derived from logarithmic graphs.

Table 1. 21 chemicals tested in a developmental toxicity test using mouse ESCs (N, non-toxicant; W, weak toxicant; M, moderate toxicant; S, strong toxicant)

No	Chemicals	CAS No.	Mw	Class	Function
1	Sodium bicarbonate	144-55-8	84.01	N	Food additive (EU, E500)
2	Sodium gluconate	527-07-01	218.14	N	Chelating agent
3	Saccharin	82385-42-0	205.17	N	artificial sweetener
4	Penicillin G	113-98-4	372.48	N	Antibiotic
5	Isoniazid	54-85-3	137.14	N	Antibiotic, Initial therapy of active tuberculosis
6	Ascorbic acid	134-03-2	198.11	N	Antioxidant
7	Doxylamine succinate	562-10-7	388.46	W	Antihistamine, Antiallergy
8	Pravastatin	81131-70-6	446.51	W	Hypocholesterolemic drug
9	Caffeine	58-08-2	194.19	W	Psychoactive drug, natural pesticide
10	Aspirin	50-78-2	180.16	W	Non-steroidal, Anti-inflammatory
11	Diphenhydramine	147-24-0	291.82	M	Antihistamine, Antiallergy, Antiemetic
12	Diphenylhydantoin	57-41-0	252.27	M	Anti-seizure
13	Indomethacin	53-86-1	357.79	M	Non-steroidal, Anti-inflammatory
14	Dexamethasone	50-02-2	392.46	M	Steroidal, Anti-inflammatory, Anti-Rheumatic
15	Papaverine	61-25-6	375.85	M	Opium alkaloid antispasmodic drug
16	Lovastatin	75330-75-5	404.54	M	Hypocholesterolemic drug
17	Verapamil-HCl	152-11-4	491.06	M	Calcium channel blocker, Antiarrhythmic agent
18	Methotrexate	133073-73-1	454.44	S	Abortifacient, Anti-Rheumatic, Antitumor
19	D-Penicillamine	52-67-5	149.21	S	Chelating agent
20	Ochratoxin A	303-47-9	403.81	S	Toxin produced by Aspergillus ochraceus
21	Retinoic Acid	302-79-4	300.44	S	Metabolite of vitamin A (retinol)

Results

Exposure to toxicants resulted in increased cell death and reduced EB area in mouse ESCs. Tested chemicals were roughly categorized based on their typical concentration-response curves obtained for EB area and the viability of ESCs and 3T3 cells over the tested concentration range of each test chemicals. Strongly embryotoxic chemicals including methotrexate, ochratoxin-A, and retinoic acid inhibited growth and differentiation of EBs and showed a high cytotoxicity to 3T3 cells and ESCs at very low concentrations. As the toxic potency of the chemical increased, the concentration at which cellular viability, growth, and differentiation rapidly decreased. The EB area was reduced in a dose-dependent manner by the tested chemicals (Fig. 1B), and a decrease in EB area resulted in a decline in beating ratio during cardiac differentiation. The 50% inhibitory concentration of EB area (ID_{50}EB) was highly correlated with the ID_{50}CM (correlation coefficient, 0.8842). Thus, the EBT can reflect not only the cytotoxicity of a chemical but also the differentiation toxicity. The developmentally toxic levels of various chemicals were evaluated and classified by using a prediction model (PM) based on IC_{50}ESC, IC_{50}3T3, and ID_{50}EB (Fig. 2A–C). To classify the chemical results into four classes, the EBT-PM included four linear functions that could best divide groups with different characteristics along a plane. Among the results of functions I, II, III, and IV of the EBT-PM, if the value of linear function I is the largest, the group is classified as non-embryotoxic. If the value of function II is largest, the toxicity is weak. If function III is largest, toxicity is moderate, and if function IV is largest, toxicity is strong (Fig. 2D).

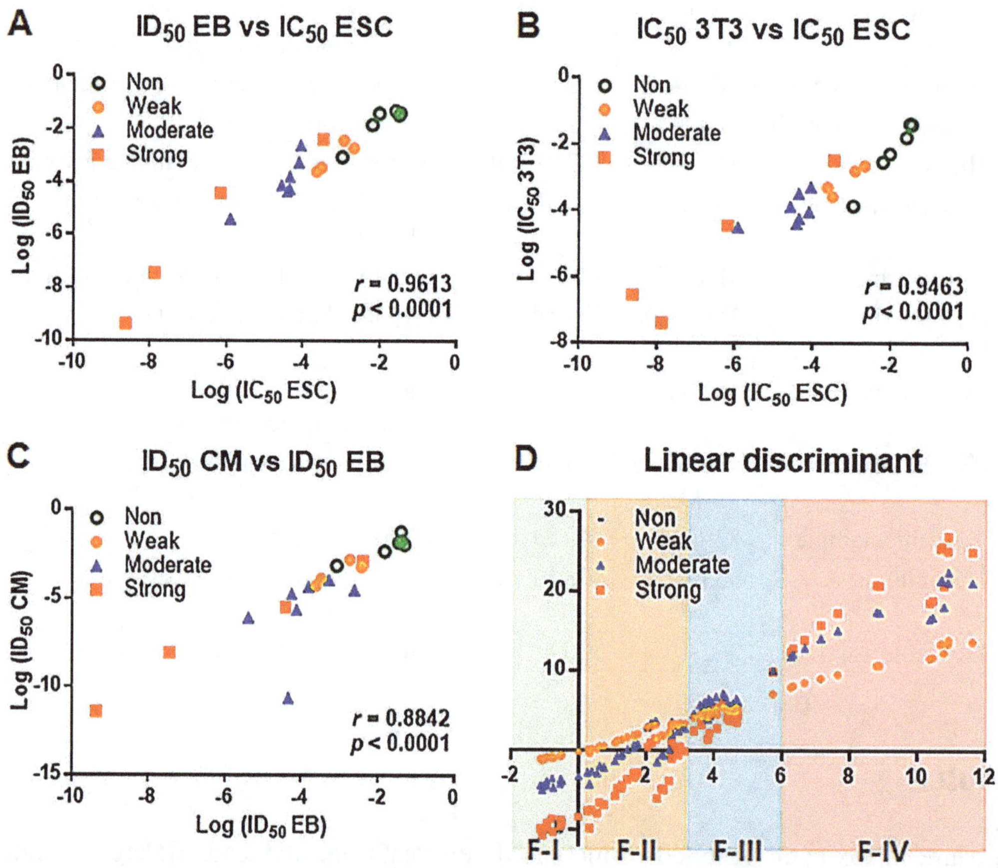

Fig. 2. Relationship between endpoints and classification for 21 chemicals. On the log scale, the correlation coefficients between (A) ID_{50}EB and IC_{50}ESC, (B) IC_{50}3T3 and IC_{50}ESC, and (C) ID_{50}CM and ID_{50}EB were 0.9613, 0.9463, and 0.8842, respectively. (D) Non-, weak, moderate, and strong toxicants were classified according to the highest value among functions I, II, III, and IV.

Discussion

The EBT assesses the developmental toxicity of chemicals at three endpoints: viability of ESCs, viability of 3T3 cells, and reduction in EB area. The three EBT endpoints were verified by performing experiments independently and repeatedly (three or more times in triplicate; 3×3). In comparison with the toxicity classification according to *in vivo* data, the EBT-PM showed a prediction accuracy of 90.5%. Developmental toxicants at toxicity-inducing concentrations resulted in a reduction in EB area and a deterioration of EB quality, which indicate the potential for growth retardation and abnormal differentiation in embryos. Chemical treatments resulted in dose-dependent decreases in the EB area via epigenetic inhibition of differentiation and arrest of the cell cycle. To determine the reliability and relevance of the EBT, a validation process is required. In this study, the initial evaluation determined that EB area assessment could be used instead of CM assessment to indicate the differentiation-related toxicity of chemicals. The EBT is a novel toxicological screening system that can facilitate rapid evaluation of embryotoxicants.

Acknowledgement. This research was supported by a grant (15182MFDS460 and 17182MFDS487) from Ministry of Food and Drug Safety in 2017.

References

1. Doke SK, Dhawale SC (2015) Alternatives to animal testing: a review. Saudi Pharm J 23 (3):223–229 SPJ: the official publication of the Saudi Pharmaceutical Society
2. Pellizzer C et al (2005) Developmental toxicity testing from animal towards embryonic stem cells. Altex 22(2):47–57
3. Adler S et al (2011) Alternative (non-animal) methods for cosmetics testing: current status and future prospects-2010. Arch Toxicol 85(5):367–485

Futuristic Approach to Alternative Model Organisms: Hydra Stakes Its Claim

Anbazhagan Murugadas[1,2], Mohammed Zeeshan[1,2], and Mohammad A. Akbarsha[1,3(✉)]

[1] Mahatma Gandhi—Doerenkamp Center for Alternatives, Bharathidasan University, Tiruchirappalli 620024, India
{biomuruga23, mdzeesh, akbarbdu}@gmail.com
[2] Department of Environmental Biotechnology, Bharathidasan University, Tiruchirappalli 620024, India
[3] National College (Autonomous), Tiruchirappalli 620001, India

Abstract. The use of mammalian models for toxicological risk assessment of chemicals has been a widespread practice for well over 50 years. This has remained controversial in view of the species differences. Further, the advances in molecular biology techniques have revolutionized the toxicological risk assessment scenario by creating demand for rapid, less expensive and highly relevant methods to risk-evaluate chemical substances quickly. In order to take advantage of these advances the US EPA funded the National Research Council to develop a strategy and vision for toxicity testing in 21st century (Tox21). Tox21 envisions a paradigm shift in toxicity testing and proposes the use of emerging technologies based on non-animal methods for better understanding of chemical-environment interaction, and also emphasizes the adoption of animals belonging to lower levels of taxonomic hierarchy, which are less sentient, in *in vivo* toxicity testing. Adoption of this shift would perhaps benefit translation of the REACH Legislation, which otherwise greatly relies on animal experiments for chemical risk assessment. We aimed at establishing *Hydra*, a simple organism belonging to Phylum Cnidaria, as a model organism for toxicity testing of environmental chemicals. Besides, *Hydra* offers advantages such as easy to culture, reproduces fast, cost-effective and highly sensitivity to inorganic pollutants. Moreover, the whole genome sequence of hydra revealed that most of the genes are conserved in which sense it offers advantage over even in the most routinely used other invertebrate model organisms. We standardized several assay methods which formed the nucleus of several publications. Herein we show that *Hydra* can be used as a viable bio-indicator for early warning of aquatic pollutants.

Keywords: *Hydra* model · Invertebrate · Toxicity testing · Budding Regeneration · ROS · Apoptosis

H. Kojima et al. (Eds.): *Alternatives to Animal Testing*, pp. 110–123, 2019.
https://doi.org/10.1007/978-981-13-2447-5_14

Introduction

Chemicals are the basic constituents of living as well as non-living things. Many chemicals naturally occur and many are synthesized. Production and/or consumption/utilization of chemical substances has increased manifold over the period of time, resulting in humans and animals getting exposed to large varieties and volumes of chemical entities directly and/or indirectly. The toxicities of many chemicals are known although thorough risk assessment has not been done for most of the chemicals. This is particularly true of many chemicals belonging to the categories such as nanoparticles and pesticides. Their fate, behavior and adverse effects are not adequately understood, particularly when they exist as mixtures (Geissen et al. 2015). These chemicals, released from the sites of industrial production and/or domestic applications and storage, are carried into the environment through contaminated water, landfill leakage and sewage effluents, and ultimately arrive at the aquatic bodies which, therefore, need special attention (Quinn et al. 2008; Patwardhan and Ghaskadbi 2013; Marchesano et al. 2015). Many chemical substances may degrade as they arrive at the aquatic environment or soon thereafter, whereas the others do not break down easily, so would enter the aquatic organisms and move up the food chain to the higher tropic levels and bio-accumulate, which is a serious threat to the aquatic biota and to the terrestrial animals, including man, which have access to the aquatic ecosystems through the food chain (Murugadas et al. 2016). In view of the adverse effects these chemical substances produce in animals and humans, the lack of knowledge about their behavior and fate, which in turn is due to paucity of sampling and/or analytical techniques, is a big issue. Therefore, multiple actions are required at various levels for risk assessment of chemical pollutants in the aquatic environment (Geissen et al. 2015).

It is generally agreed that health of the ecosystem is measured not only in terms of chemical and physical qualities of water but also in terms abundance and health of biota of the ecosystem (Herricks and Schaeffer 1985). The latter calls for testing of chemical substances per se or the polluted waters in organisms that would in their natural habitat be exposed to such chemicals. In other words, it is better that testing is done in an environmentally related species. However, while fish would fit into this slot, invertebrates should be of preference in the light of uptake of chemical entities from the aquatic environment, by direct ingestion, contaminated preys, water filtration, surface contact and inhalation (Cattaneo et al. 2009). Among the aquatic invertebrates, ones with unlimited supply, small size, simple body plan, and short life cycle, together with that are easy to maintain and cost-effective, and can better be groomed into a suitable model organism. From a regulatory perspective this is highly pertinent and relevant since the US Tox21 vision envisaged adoption of mechanistic models, including non-vertebrate organisms for hazard assessment of chemical substances (Krewski et al. 2010). More recently, the Toxic Chemical Substances Act (TSCA) 1976 of USA has been amended as the "Frank R. Lautenburg Chemical Safety for the 21st Century Act 2016." This revised law includes a new section [4 (h)], entitled Reduction of Testing on Vertebrates has been added, according to which EPA must "develop a strategic plan to promote the development and implementation of alternative test methods and strategies to reduce, refine or replace vertebrate animal testing…", implying encouragement of use of non-vertebrate models. Under these circumstances, extensive research has been undertaken in our laboratory to standardize the cnidarian polyp *Hydra* as a model organism for evaluating the aquatic eco-toxicity of chemical substances and emerging pollutants. *Hydra* is a small diploblastic organism. It is available in abundance in fresh water bodies. It reproduces profusely by budding, thereby producing identical twins. *Hydra* has also the remarkable capability to regenerate its amputated body region, making it virtually immortal. It is not known to feel pain and, therefore, does not need an ethical clearance. All cells in *Hydra* are in close proximity to and contact with the aquatic environment, which facilitates permeation of chemical substances into the animal (Beach and Pascoe 1998). In this paper we present an overview of the assay methods encompassing morpho-physiological features, feeding behavior, growth rate, regeneration, nuclear morphology, cell cycle analysis, apoptosis, and changes at molecular level endpoints for aquatic toxicity testing of chemical entities including nanomaterials.

Hydra-Systematics

Hydra is a fresh water eumetazoan diploblastic organism belonging to Phylum Cnidaria, Class Hydrozoa, Order Anthomedusae/Anthoathecata, and Family Hydroidea. The body is a cylindrical polyp which is radial. It is essentially a sedentary organism living attached to stones, pebbles and water plants, but can get released from the substratum and swim.

Physiology and Anatomy

Hydra measures about 10–15 mm long when fully extended. It is cylindrical and tubular. The oral end of the body column consists of conical hypostome, surrounded by 3–10 tentacles which play role in prey capture, and the aboral end consists of basal disc with which it attaches to the substratum. The body column is divided into four distinctive regions, (i) the gastric region which extends between the tentacle and the first apical bud, where it digests the prey; (ii) the budding section, which produces the bud; (iii) the peduncle, located between the lowest bud and the basal disc; and (iv) the foot region (Hecker and Slobodkin 1976) (Fig. 1). The body wall is comprised of an outer ectoderm or epidermis and an inner endoderm or gastrodermis, both of which are formed of epithelio-muscular cells, separated by a non-cellular jelly-like mesoglea. There is a primitive form of nervous system consisting of a net of neurons underlying the epidermis, as well as gastrodermis. Cells unique to cnidarians – the cnidoblasts or nematocytes, with a toxin-laden nematocyst inside – are very specialized, and engage in offence and defense, playing a role in feeding by paralyzing the prey. *Hydra* consists of three different stem cell lineages, including ectodermal and endodermal epithelial cell lineages, which self-renew by continuous division and migrate towards both the extremities and terminally differentiate. The third stem cell lineage consists of interstitial cells which are multipotent and can differentiate into neurons, secretory cells and gametes. In view of the effectively dividing and expanding stem cell lineages, *Hydra* is practically an immortal organism.

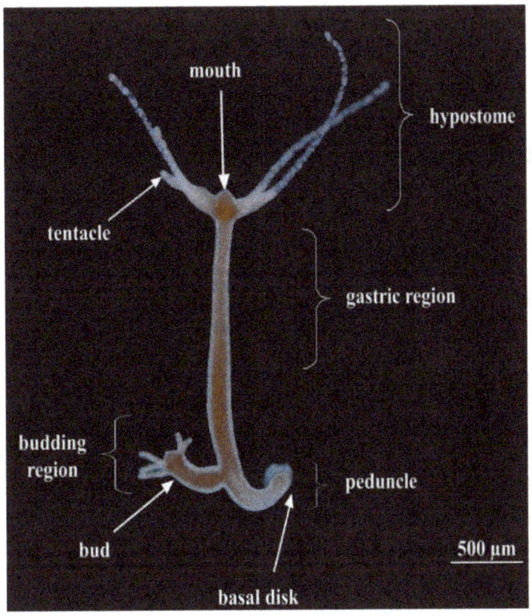

Fig. 1. Morphology of *Hydra*

Reproduction

Hydra can reproduce by both sexual and asexual methods. The primary form of reproduction is asexual, by budding, which happens as long as conditions are favorable. Budding results in rapid production of a large number of genetically identical *Hydra*s. This genetic identity enables the researchers to reproduce experimental results with less statistical difference (Beach and Pascoe 1998). Growth rate in *Hydra* is in equilibrium state between cell proliferation and removal of excess cell by phagocytosis or bud formation (Bosch and David 1984). However, during unfavorable condition or in the context of environmental contamination, the growth rate is affected, and the animal engages in sexual reproduction resulting in cysts that can endure adverse conditions (Ambrosone et al. 2014).

Regeneration

Hydra is known for its remarkable capability of regeneration. Amputation of *Hydra* into any number of pieces other than hypostome and basal disc can result in each such piece regenerating the missing parts. It has been stated that *Hydra* undergoes morphallactic regeneration to restore its unique structure after amputation (Bode 2003). In case of head regeneration, wound healing occurs in 3–6 h, the tentacles begin to emerge within 30–36 h, and complete head regeneration occurs within 48–72 h of amputation. Similarly, in case of foot regeneration, epithelial cells extend to heal the wound site and the foot regenerates approximately in 30 h. This dynamic process of regeneration in *Hydra* is tightly regulated by specific genes. Methods have been developed to quantify the abnormal morphologies as well as alterations in gene expression in *Hydra* following exposure to an environmental stress, which render *Hydra* recognized as the ideal model organism to test teratogenicity of environmental pollutants (Wilby 1988; Ambrosone et al. 2014).

End Point Analysis

Morphological Observation in *Hydra* Following Exposure to Chemicals

Toxicity testing in *Hydra* is manifested by alterations in its morphology, starting with contraction of tentacles and shortening of body column and ending up in animal disintegration. The scoring system for *Hydra*'s morphology was originally designed by Johnson and Gabel (1983), and later improved by Wilby (1988). Thereafter, Wilby's scale of toxicity testing has served as the basis for the determination of toxicity of chemical compounds in *Hydra* from the perspective of morphological changes. As toxicant concentration increases, progressive changes occur in *Hydra*'s morphology. A score of 10 was assigned to highly intact and healthy polyps, 8 to clubbed tentacles, 6 to shortened tentacles, 5 to tulip phase, 3 and 2 to osmoregulation loss, and 0 to animals that had undergone disintegration (Table 1; Fig. 2). Recently, Ambrosone et al. (2014) observed different phenotypic variations in *Hydra* when treated with SiO_2 nanoparticles, based on which a new scaling system to assess the detrimental effects of nanoparticles in *Hydra* was devised (Table 2).

Table 1. Scoring system devised by Wilby (1988) for assessing the morphological damage following toxicant exposure.

Score	Morphology of polyp
10	Extended tentacles; body reactive
9	Partially contracted; slow reactions
8	Clubbed tentacles; body slightly contracted
7	Shortened tentacles; body slightly contracted
6	Tentacles and body shortened
5	Totally contracted; tentacles visible
4	Totally contracted; no visible tentacles
3	Expanded; tentacles visible
2	Expanded; no visible tentacles
1	Dead but intact
0	Disintegrated

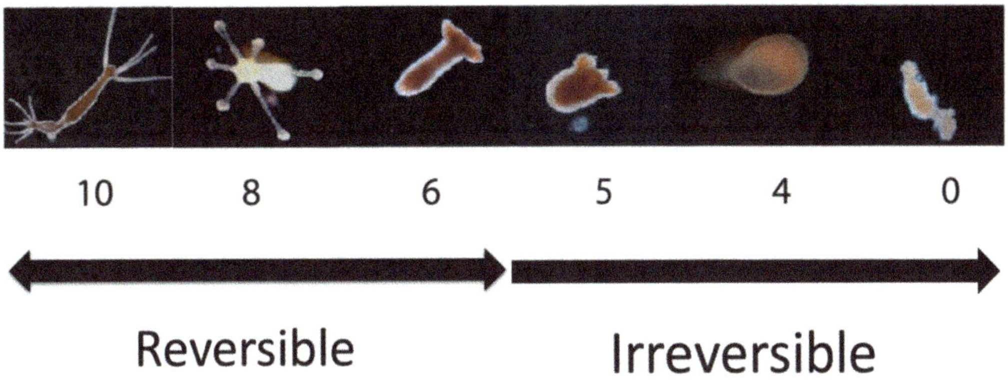

Fig. 2. Representation of Wilby's (1988) scale of toxicity testing for assessing the morphological damage following toxicant exposure. (Adopted from: Murugadas et al. 2016).

Table 2. Scoring system devised by Ambrosone et al. (2014) to measure the morphological traits in hydra following nanoparticle exposure

Score	Morphology	Vital state
7	Normal hydra	Active
6	Bumped gastric regions, normal tentacles	Active
5	Inverted-cone gastric regions, shortened tentacles	Whitening of gastric region; paralyzed, slow tentacles
4	Inverted-cone gastric regions, short tentacles	Paralyzed, rigid tentacles
3	Gastric region reduced in size, crushed tentacles	Permanently damaged to death
2	Further reduced gastric region, without tentacles	Abundant cell death
1	Irregular shape	Death
0	Dispersed cell clamps and debris	Disintegrated

Methodology

For aquatic eco-toxicity testing, *Hydra* is placed at one per mL of medium (1 mM $CaCl_2$, 1 mM NaCl, 0.1 mM $MgSO_4$, 0.1 mM KCl, and 1 mM Tris-HCl; pH 7.8). Depending on the container capacity, a minimum of 10–25 animals are taken for each experiment, and care is taken to pick those animals which do not possess bud or with only slightly developed bud, to avoid increase in the number of animals at the end of the experiment. For a controlled laboratory experiment, the polyps should be maintained at 18 ± 1 °C under 12 h dark-light cycle. The experiment can be initiated by adding varying concentrations of the chemical substance to the culture dishes and monitoring continuously in a stereo-zoom microscope throughout the study period (72 or 96 h). The morphological variations are recorded at regular time intervals. Animals that respond in a specific time are assigned with a median score for determination of median lethal concentration. A score of 5 or less is considered to be lethal and the change is irreversible; in the case of score above 5 the change is reversible, wherein the animal becomes healthy when healthy environment is restored. For a concentration- and/or time-dependent toxicity, the median score is indirectly proportional to the incubation time and concentration tested.

Impact of Chemicals on *Hydra* Growth Rate

Hydra primarily reproduces by budding, which is an asexual method of reproduction. The extent of budding is directly related to food intake. A regular diet maintains the cell proliferation and budding process, whereas budding ceases when starved. In view of a regular feeding regime, the epithelial cell lineage that migrates towards both extremities contributes to bud formation in the gastric region. Thus, growth rate of *Hydra* is a balance between length of epithelial cell cycle, phagocytosis of the excess cells, and/or bud formation (Bosch and David 1984). Quality of the environment, including chemical contamination, affects the growth rate in *Hydra* (Lenhoff and Brown 1970).

Methodology

To measure the growth rate of *Hydra*, four *Hydra*s each with one bud are exposed to sub-lethal doses of chemical entities for a study period (24 h in case of acute toxicity), and then washed and placed in multi-well plates, preferably as one *Hydra* per well. Control polyps at the same developmental stage are left untreated and maintained separately. Both treated and untreated *Hydra*s are fed regularly atleast for two weeks and monitored every day for bud detachment. The growth rate constant (K) is measured using the formula $K = \ln (n/n_0)/T$, where n is the number of animals at time T (day of experiment), n_0 is the number animals at time t_0, i.e., starting day of the experiment; budding rate is calculated as the average number of buds detached per *Hydra* per day; T2, the population doubling time, is calculated by linear regression (Ambrosone et al. 2012).

Impact of Chemicals on *Hydra's* Regeneration Ability

Hydra is known for remarkable capability of regenerating missing body parts. *Hydra* undergoes morphallactic regeneration where the tissue left over in a bisected region is remodeled to regenerate the missing body structure. Though *Hydra* has three different cell lineages, regeneration is taken care by the two epithelial cell lineages. Head regeneration is rapid after bisection of the tubular body column, wherein complete regeneration occurs within 72 h.

Teratogenicity testing in *Hydra* was initially described by Johnson and Gabel (1983) using dissociated cells of *Hydra*. Later, Wilby (1988) recommended a new scale to measure the regeneration of *Hydra* using gastric region. More recently, Ambrosone et al. (2012) proposed a new scale to measure head regeneration in *Hydra* in the presence of nanoparticles. Here, in the present review, we have summarized the methods of Ambrosone et al. (2012), and Wilby (1988) to measure the regeneration capability of *Hydra*.

Methodology

(i) Ambrosone et al. (2012): To measure the effect of toxicant on *Hydra's* head regeneration capability, groups of polyps are bisected in the upper gastric region and the body column is allowed to regenerate the missing head region in the presence of sub-lethal concentrations of the toxicant. Polyps that undergo head regeneration are examined in a stereo-zoom dissecting microscope at regular time intervals for 72 h, and

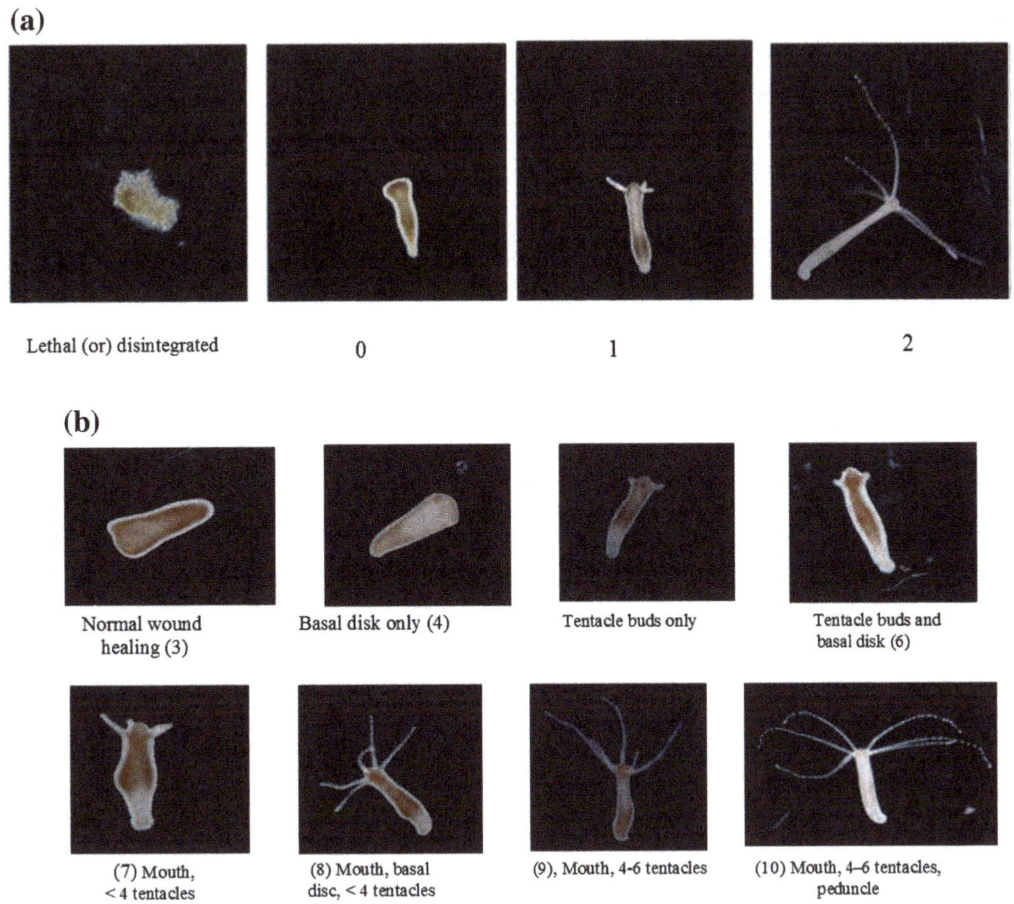

Fig. 3. a. *Hydra* images representing the scoring system devised by Ambrosone et al. (2012) to measure the head regeneration in hydra (Adopted from Murugadas et al. 2016). b. *Hydra* images representing the scoring system devised by Wilby (1988) for assessing the toxicant induced inhibition of regeneration of gastric region. (Adopted from Zeeshan et al. 2016)

Table 3. Scoring system devised by Ambrosone et al. (2012) to measure the head regeneration in hydra

Score	Degree of regeneration
0	Lethal or disintegrated
1	No regeneration
2	Emergence of tentacles
3	Complete head regeneration

score is assigned based on the regeneration. As seen in Fig. 3a and Table 3, score 0 stands for no regeneration, 1 for emergence of tentacles, 2 for complete head regeneration; lethal and disintegration can also be observed.

(ii) Wilby (1988): To measure the chronic toxic effect of a toxicant on *Hydra* regeneration, groups of polyps are cut below the hypostome and above the budding region to separate the gastric region, and allowed to regenerate the missing body portion in the presence of sub-lethal concentrations of the chemical to be tested and the medium is renewed daily. Initially, the wound healing occurs within 3–6 h and the emergence of tentacles and basal disc occurs within 36–48 h. The regeneration is recorded at every 24 h until 72 h of amputation. Score of 10 indicates complete regeneration and 0 represents mortality; scores from 9 to 1 express various stages of regeneration (Fig. 3b; Table 4).

Table 4. Scoring system of Wilby (1988) for assessing the toxicant-induced inhibition of regeneration of gastric region

Score	Degree of regeneration
10	Mouth, 4–6 tentacles and peduncle
9	Mouth, 4–6 tentacles
8	Mouth, <4 tentacles and basal disc
7	Mouth and <4 tentacles
6	Tentacle buds and basal disc
5	Tentacle buds only
4	Basal disc only
3	Normal wound healing at both ends of gastric region
2	Healed but body expanded
1	Open ends of gastric region/dissected region; not healed or dead
0	Disintegrated

However, in most cases, impairment of regeneration in *Hydra* at sub-lethal concentrations is due to the general toxicity as the chemicals/nanoparticle (NPs) can easily gain access into the *Hydra* cells via nick at either ends and induce toxicity by increasing the ROS level or sudden exposure of amputated region to a high concentration of chemicals/NPs can induce cell death.

Impact of Chemicals on *Hydra* Cell Cycle

Hydra as a whole organism possesses different cell types from three different lineages (Siebert et al. 2008). The cell cycle of interstitial cells is shorter than that of the epithelial cells. However, both cell lineages exhibit a similar regulation of cell cycle with a pause in G2 phase and lack of G1 phase (Buzgariu et al. 2014). Pausing of G2 makes *Hydra* a potential model to study the impact of pausing of G2 impinging on regenerative competence. Two major challenging tasks in analyzing the cell cycle of a multicellular organism are, (i) to dissociate the complex cell types into individual cells, and (ii) to sort the cells of a similar type based on the marker genes. Cell cycle analysis overcoming these challenges is still possible, taking advantage of the latest advancements in technologies, and it helps in determining the detrimental effects of chemical entities and also in designing new drugs.

Methodology
The simplest and most convenient way to dissociate *Hydra* is to adopt trypsin digestion. After incubation with the toxicant *Hydras* are rinsed in fresh medium and dissociated in 250 μL of trypsin-EDTA for 5–7 min at 37 °C. Trypsin is inactivated by addition of 100 μL of fetal calf serum (FCS) to the cell suspension. The cells, at $5 * 10^5$/mL, are fixed in 4% paraformaldehyde and permeabilized using 70% ethanol. Cells are then stained with 500 μL of hypertonic NP-40 buffer [Propidium Iodide (PI)] 40 μg/mL, RNase A 200 μg/mL, 0.5% NP-40 in PBS), for 15–30 min. The fluorescence emission is measured (Buzgariu et al. 2014) on a FACS Calibur II System (Becton–Dickinson) using an argon-ion laser at 488 nm, together with the forward scattered (FSC) and side scattered (SSC) parameters. The emitted PI fluorescence is collected by a 585 nm band pass filter in the FL2 channel. Typically 10,000 events per sample are collected using the Cell Quest software, and analyzed with FlowJo software (Tree Star Inc) after excluding debris, clumps (FSC versus SSC) and doublets (signal area FL2-A versus signal width FL2-W).

Assessment of Cell Death in *Hydra* by ROS Generation and Apoptosis

Owing to the continuous proliferation of stem cells, excess or dead cells from *Hydra* are sloughed off by the programmed cell death, i.e. "apoptosis". It is well established that in *Hydra* apoptotic mode of cell death is conserved (Böttger and Alexandrova 2007). Therefore, *Hydra* is emerging as an appropriate model organism for drug discovery and biomedical applications. Apoptosis is induced by treatment with chemical substances or under stressful conditions. Oxidative stress sets in as a consequence of imbalance between generation of ROS triggered by external factors and the counteracting antioxidants in the biological system. Excess ROS cause DNA damage and failure of DNA repair mechanism and finally ends up in cell death.

Determination of ROS Generation in Hydra by H_2-DCFDA Staining
Groups of 6 animals per 6 mL are incubated in medium containing sub-lethal concentrations of the chemical substance to be tested, for the defined period, after which the animals are washed in fresh *Hydra* medium and incubated with 10 μM H_2-DCFDA dye for 1 h in dark as described by Jantzen et al. (1998). After incubation the polyps are rinsed in *Hydra* medium, mounted on 2% urethane, and the green punctae are observe immediately in a fluorescent microscope. For quantification of intracellular ROS level, cell lysate is prepared by homogenizing the *Hydra* in PBS. Protein concentration of the cell lysate is determined using Bradford reagent, with bovine serum albumin (BSA) as the standard. Intracellular ROS level is determined by incubating the cell lysate with 10 μM H_2-DCFDA dye for 20 min in dark and the fluorescence is read in a fluorometer.

Determination of Apoptosis by Acridine Orange and DAPI Staining

Acridine Orange Staining

Induction of apoptosis at whole animal level can be identified by acridine orange staining as described by Cikala et al. (1999). Groups of 6 animals per 6 mL are incubated in medium containing sub-lethal concentrations of the toxicants to be tested, for the defined period. After incubation polyps are rinsed in *Hydra* medium and incubated with acridine orange (3.3 μM) for 15 min in dark. Polyps are washed adequately with *Hydra* medium, relaxed in 2% urethane and the green punctae as apoptotic cells are observed in fluorescent microscope.

4′-6-Diamidino-2-Phenylindole (DAPI) Staining

Apoptosis as single cells in *Hydra* can be enumerated following DAPI staining as described by Ambrosone et al. (2012). Groups of 6 animals per 6 mL are incubated in medium containing sub-lethal concentrations of chemicals for the defined period. Single cell suspensions are prepared by macerating the *Hydra*s and spreading them on gelatin-coated microscopic slides. After adequate wash in PBS the cell suspensions are stained with DAPI for 2 min and washed in PBS. Cells are examined in a phase contrast fluorescent microscope. Cells, 300–500, are examined for each treatment and the percentage of apoptosis is calculated for both the untreated and treated cells. The comparison is necessary since cells in untreated *Hydra* also would undergo apoptosis towards maintenance of cell number.

Genotoxicity Assessment in *Hydra* Following Chemical Exposure

Genotoxicity assessment in an aquatic invertebrate organism would take it to the level of a good bio-indicator. Chemical substances that affect DNA have serious implications in many pathological conditions such as carcinogenesis and impairment of reproduction. Genotoxicity assessment in a multicellular organism is a challenging task as the organism contains many cell types of different origins. We embarked on dissociation of toxicant-exposed *Hydra* into individual cells and address the implications of chemical/nanoparticle on DNA in individual cells.

Methodology

*Hydra*s are treated with sub-lethal concentrations of the intended chemical for the specific period. *Hydra* could be dissociated into individual cells using trypsin-EDTA or homogenization using a micropipette. In our experience, effective dissociation is possible in trypsin-EDTA digestion (Murugadas et al. 2016). The resulting cell suspension is mixed with low melting agarose in PBS, and placed on microscopic slides coated with normal melting agarose. The slides are placed in pre-chilled lysis buffer (2.5 M NaCl, 100 mM Na2-EDTA, 10 mM Tris, 0.2 mM NaOH [pH 10], 10% DMSO and Triton X-100) and incubated overnight at 4 °C. Alkaline denaturation and gel electrophoresis are performed in cold under dim light in freshly prepared electrophoresis buffer (300 mM NaOH, 1 mM Na2-EDTA, [pH > 13]) for 20 min at 20 V. Then the slides are washed with neutralization buffer (0.4 M Tris, pH 7.5) and observed in fluorescent microscope. Three hundred cells from each treatment group are captured and analyzed using CASP software. The extent of DNA damage is measured according as depicted in Fig. 4 and Table 5.

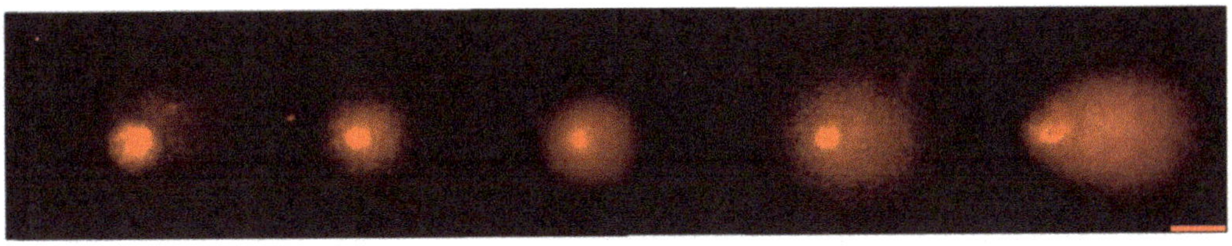

Fig. 4. Images representing the extent of DNA damage as assessed by Comet assay. (Adopted from Zeeshan et al. 2017)

Table 5. Allocation of empirical scores to cells (categorization of DNA damage and score allocation)

Percentage of DNA damage	Category assigned	Score allocated
0–5	Zero	0
6–20	Low	1
21–40	Medium	2
41–95	High	3
96–100	Complete	4

Transcriptional Alterations in *Hydra* Following Chemicals Exposure

It is well demonstrated that chemicals/heavy metals/nanoparticles can interact with nucleic acids and induce DNA damage and point mutations and alter transcriptional regulation of important genes governing antioxidant defense system and cell death (Woo et al. 2012; Murugadas et al. 2016; Zeeshan et al. 2016, 2017). The whole genome sequencing of *Hydra* has revealed that it has conserved sequences and signaling pathways of divergent organisms and makes it comparable with the other model organisms. Thus, toxicant-exposed Hydras can be subjected to RNA isolation, cDNA synthesis and qPCR to assess the transcriptional alterations, which we intend to standardize and bring out in our next review.

Conclusion

In view of varied manifestations of emerging pollutants, risk assessment of the chemical entities before releasing them into the environment is necessary. *Hydra* as a model organism is easy to culture, multiplies rapidly by asexual reproduction, cost-effective, sensitive to inorganic substances, morphological changes can be easily monitored and classified, and genetically identical twins can be made use of for reproducible results at transcriptional levels. Its robust nature of whole body regeneration from the dissociated cells or gastric region or body column makes *Hydra* a suitable organism for teratogenicity testing. A comprehensive study including various end point analyses and expression of biomarker genes can explain the underlying mechanism of toxicity induced by various chemical substances. Thus, *Hydra* is an organism highly suited for aquatic eco-toxicity testing.

Acknowledgments. The financial support from Doerenkamp-Zbinden Foundation, Switzerland, is heartily acknowledged.

References

Ambrosone A, Mattera L, Marchesano V et al (2012) Mechanisms underlying toxicity induced by CdTe quantum dots determined in an invertebrate model organism. Biomaterials 33 (7):1991–2000. https://doi.org/10.1016/j.biomaterials.2011.11.041

Ambrosone A, Scotto di Vettimo MR, Malvindi MA et al (2014) Impact of amorphous SiO_2 nanoparticles on a living organism: Morphological, behavioral, and molecular biology implications. Front Bioeng Biotechnol 2:37. https://doi.org/10.3389/fbioe.2014.00037

Beach MJ, Pascoe D (1998) Therole of *Hydra vulgaris* (Pallas) in assessing the toxicity of freshwater pollutants. Water Res 32(1):101–106. https://doi.org/10.1016/S0043-1354(97)00180-2

Bode HR (2003) Head regeneration in Hydra. Dev Dyn 226(2):225–236. https://doi.org/10.1002/dvdy.10225

Bosch TCG, David CN (1984) Growth regulation in Hydra: relationship between epithelial cell cycle length and growth rate. Dev Biol 104(1):161–171. https://doi.org/10.1016/0012-1606(84)90045-9

Böttger A, Alexandrova O (2007) Programmed cell death in Hydra. Sem Cancer Biol 17(2):134–146. https://doi.org/10.1016/j.semcancer.2006.11.008

Buzgariu W, Crescenzi M, Galliot B (2014) Robust G2 pausing of adult stem cells in Hydra. Differentiation 87(1):83–99. https://doi.org/10.1016/j.diff.2014.03.001

Cattaneo A, Gornati R, Chiriva-Internati M, Bernardini G (2009) Ecotoxicology of nanomaterials: the role of invertebrate testing. Exposure 6:78–97

Cikala M, Wilm B, Hobmayer E, Böttger A, David CN (1999) Identification of caspases and apoptosis in the simple metazoan Hydra. Curr Biol 9(17):959–962. https://doi.org/10.1016/S0960-9822(99)80423-0

Geissen V, Mol H, Klumpp E et al (2015) Emerging pollutants in the environment: a challenge for water resource management. Int Soil Water Conserv Res 3(1):57–65. https://doi.org/10.1016/j.iswcr.2015.03.002

Hecker B, Slobodkin LB (1976) Responses of *Hydra oligactis* to temperature and feeding rate. In: Mackie GO (ed) Coelenterate ecology and behavior. Springer, Boston, MA, pp 175–183. https://doi.org/10.1007/978-1-4757-9724-4_19

Herricks EE, Schaeffer DJ (1985) Can we optimize biomonitoring? Environ Manag 9(6):487–492. https://doi.org/10.1007/bf01867323

Jantzen H, Hassel M, Schulze I (1998) Hydroperoxides mediate lithium effects on regeneration in *Hydra*. Comp Biochem Physiol C Pharmacol Toxicol Endocrinol 119(2):165–175. https://doi.org/10.1016/S0742-8413(97)00204-1

Johnson EM, Gabel BEG (1983) An artificial 'Embryo' for detection of abnormal developmental biology. Fundam Appl Toxicol 3(4):243–249. https://doi.org/10.1016/S0272-0590(83)80135-3

Krewski D, Acosta D, Andersen M et al (2010) Toxicity testing in the 21st century: a vision and a strategy. J Toxicol Env Health B Critical Rev 13:51–138. https://doi.org/10.1080/10937404.2010.483176

Lenhoff HM, Brown RD (1970) Mass culture of Hydra: an improved method and its application to other aquatic invertebrates. Lab Anim 4(1):139–154. https://doi.org/10.1258/002367770781036463

Marchesano V, Ambrosone A, Bartelmess J et al (2015) Impact of carbon nano-onions on *Hydra vulgaris* as a model organism for nanoecotoxicology. Nanomaterials 5(3):1331–1350

Murugadas A, Zeeshan M, Thamaraiselvi K, Ghaskadbi S, Akbarsha MA (2016) Hydra as a model organism to decipher the toxic effects of copper oxide nanorod: eco-toxicogenomics approach. Sci Rep 6:29663. https://doi.org/10.1038/srep29663

Patwardhan V, Ghaskadbi S (2013) Invertebrate alternatives for toxicity testing: hydra stakes its claim. Altex Proc 2(1):69–76

Quinn B, Gagné F, Blaise C (2008) The effects of pharmaceuticals on the regeneration of the cnidarian, Hydra attenuata. Sci Total Environ 402(1):62–69. https://doi.org/10.1016/j.scitotenv.2008.04.039

Siebert S, Anton-Erxleben F, Bosch TCG (2008) Cell type complexity in the basal metazoan Hydra is maintained by both stem cell based mechanisms and trans differentiation. Dev Biol 313(1):13–24. https://doi.org/10.1016/j.ydbio.2007.09.007

Wilby OK (1988) The Hydra regeneration assay. In: Proceedings of Assoc Francaise de Teratologie, pp 108–124

Woo S, Lee A, Won H, Ryu J-C, Yum S (2012) Toxaphene affects the levels of mRNA transcripts that encode antioxidant enzymes in Hydra. Comp Biochem Physiol C Toxicol Pharmacol 156(1):37–41. https://doi.org/10.1016/j.cbpc.2012.03.005

Zeeshan M, Murugadas A, Ghaskadbi S, Rajendran BR, Akbarsha MA (2016) ROS dependent copper toxicity in Hydra- Biochemical and molecular study. Comp Biochem Physiol C Toxicol Pharmacol 185–186(Supplement C):1–12. doi:https://doi.org/10.1016/j.cbpc.2016.02.008

Zeeshan M, Murugadas A, Ghaskadbi S, Ramaswamy BR, Akbarsha MA (2017) Ecotoxicological assessment of cobalt using Hydra model: ROS, oxidative stress, DNA damage, cell cycle arrest, and apoptosis as mechanisms of toxicity. Environ Pollut 224(Supplement C):54–69. doi:https://doi.org/10.1016/j.envpol.2016.12.042

The Lush Prize and Young Researcher Asia Awards 2016

Rebecca Ram(✉)

Clinical Data Scientist and Scientific Research Consultant-Lush Prize, London, UK
rebecca@lushprize.org
http://lushprize.org

Abstract. The Lush Prize is now in its fifth year and awards a total of 52,000,000 JPY (approx.) annually to initiatives working to end the use of animals in toxicology testing. There are six categories of award: Science; Training; Young Researcher; Lobbying and Public Awareness. The sixth category is the Lush Black Box Prize which offers, in any one year, a further 38,000,000 JPY (approx.) for a key breakthrough in human toxicology. Many initiatives are directed at the '3Rs': reduction, refinement, and replacement of the use of animals. The Lush Prize seeks only to support projects working on the genuine replacement of animal tests and is the largest reward in its field [1].

In 2016, the Prize is very pleased to announce the launch of its Young Researcher Asia awards, to welcome young scientists from across Asia, up to 35 years old at time of application, who wish to pursue a career in animal-free toxicology. Applicants complete a nomination explaining their research proposals, including how they would use a bursary of approx. 1,400,000 JPY. To date in 2016, a total of 37,800,000 JPY has been awarded to nineteen international young researchers for 21st century human-relevant toxicology projects.

The Lush Prize continues to welcome nominations from across the Asia region, not only for Young Researcher awards, but all other prize categories. This report aims to provide an overview of the Prize, the categories of award available, achievements to date and further background information.

Introduction

The Lush Prize was developed to address two urgent goals; firstly, to fund the development of modern, more reliable methods of human-relevant safety testing and secondly but equally importantly, to replace unreliable and inhumane animal tests.

Many scientists find that access to funding for research into non-animal technologies can be a barrier. The Lush Prize wants to change this and encourage young researchers to develop a career in toxicology without harming animals, by offering bursaries to allow them to advance in this area. The Lush Prize is now in its fifth year and awards an annual total of 52,000,000 JPY (approx.) to initiatives working to end the use of animals in toxicology testing. There are six categories of award: Science; Training; Young Researcher; Lobbying and Public Awareness. The sixth category is

H. Kojima et al. (Eds.): *Alternatives to Animal Testing*, pp. 124–128, 2019.
https://doi.org/10.1007/978-981-13-2447-5_15

the Lush Black Box Prize which offers, in any one year, a further 38,000,000 JPY (approx.) for a key breakthrough in human toxicology. An overview of the different categories is provided below.

The Lush Prize Categories

1. Science - For individuals, research teams or institutions for work conducted on relevant toxicity pathways. Outstanding research producing an effective non-animal safety test based on an approach other than toxicity pathways, where none existed before, may also be considered.
2. Young Researchers - Open to scientists (up to 35 years of age at the time of application) with a desire to fund the next stage of a career in animal free toxicology. (The annual YR prize fund is usually divided between five winners, each awarded approx 1,400,000 JPY). The Young Researcher prizes are distinct from other categories as they awarded on the basis of *future* research proposals, intended to replace the use of animals. All other categories of prize are awarded on the basis of *past* activities and achievements, over the previous 12–18 months.

The Science and Young Researcher Prizes are designed to advance direct research into non-animal technologies. The Lush Prize is pleased to launch the Young Researcher Asia Awards at the 2016 JSAAE Congress.

3. Training - For individuals, teams or organisations involved in training others in non-animal methods. There remains an ongoing, urgent need for education and training in the use of widely available, human-relevant, non-animal technologies; communication on this is vital and remains an obstacle to change. Many establishments or individuals may not have been trained in available, animal-free methods or might not even be aware of them, while future scientists and students need to be provided with education in alternative methods, in order to be able to pursue further research in this area. This prize recognises the importance of relevant information and hands-on training among commercial scientists, researchers and students.

The Training Prize is designed to aid resource for projects training scientists or regulators in non-animal methods.

4. Lobbying - The Lobbying prize rewards exceptional individuals, groups or organisations pushing for change, focusing on policy interventions promoting the replacement or end of animal tests. These may include science-based lobbying at national or international level, for example to recognise non-animal testing methods in national or international (e.g. Organisation for Economic and Cooperative Development (OECD) programmes of test guidelines [2], removal of animal tests and achieving mandatory requirements for non-animal methods in legislation, regulatory policies and testing guidelines.
5. Public Awareness - Organisations and individuals working to raise awareness on both the ongoing suffering associated with animal testing and the scientific need for

its replacement are recognised by the Public Awareness prize. Winners are awarded for their work in ensuring that these issues remain high on the public agenda.

The Public Awareness and Lobbying Prizes are designed to maintain pressure and influence, to ensure regulation is updated to reflect advances in 21st-Century toxicology.

The Black Box Prize

A special sixth category of prize is the Black Box Prize. It may offer a full 38,000 000 JPY (approx.) in any one year, for a key breakthrough in research into pathways of human toxicity in response to chemicals, replacing the use of animals.

The first Black Box prize was awarded in 2015, to several individuals and organisations for their achievements in the development of new in-vitro test methods which elucidated the Adverse Outcome Pathway (AOP) for skin sensitisation, now accepted at OECD level [3].

The Lush Prize Is a '1R' Initiative

Many funding schemes are devoted to 'the 3Rs'; Reduction, Refinement, Replacement of the use of animals in experiments. However, as 'reduction' and 'refinement' methods still involve animals, the Lush Prize only supports projects working towards the '1R'- the complete replacement of animal tests. It is the largest prize fund in the world devoted to this initiative.

Launch of Lush Prize 'Young Researcher Asia' Awards in 2016

In 2016, the Prize is very pleased to announce the launch of its Young Researcher Asia Awards and welcomes young scientists from across Asia, up to 35 years old at time of application, who wish to pursue a career in animal-free toxicology. Applicants complete a nomination explaining their research proposals, including how they would use a bursary of approx. 1,400,000 JPY. To date in 2016, a total of 37,800,000 JPY has been awarded to nineteen international young researchers for human-relevant toxicology projects. Our 2016 Young Researcher Award winning projects [4] include research themes of;

- Development of innovative 3D human skin models to test cosmetics
- Human tissue-derived test methods to assess how chemicals cause hepatotoxicity
- Establishment of human based *in vitro* methods to test dental and medical devices.

Projects Funded by the Lush Prize to Date

- 8 international scientific organisations for projects including human lung cancer tissue culture models, body-on-a chip systems, 'omics' technology-derived data from analysis of human in-vitro and in-silico models, QSARs (Quantitative Structure Activity Relationships) and work on toxicity pathways in heptatoxicity and developmental toxicity.

- 32 young researchers and early career scientists from across the world, with bursaries totalling more than 40,000,000 JPY.
- 8 outstanding Training prize winning organisations, for projects including preparation and delivery of training workshops and webinars, outreach and communication in universities and educational establishments across the world and direct delivery of 'hands-on' training in non-animal methods in China.
- 11 Public Awareness projects (total more than 45,000,000 JPY) for breakthrough investigational campaigns highlighting the suffering of non-human primates, cats and dogs; initiatives to end toxicity testing in the USA, Switzerland, China, Russia, Canada and Japan and finally, campaigns on banning animal tested cosmetics in Taiwan, Australia and New Zealand.
- 10 Policy makers, political figures and scientific organisations devoted to alternatives to animal testing from the USA, Sweden, Germany, New Zealand, Brazil and India have been awarded more than 45,000,000 JPY in Lobbying Prize funding to date.

Since its launch in 2012, the Lush Prize has awarded over 210,000,000 JPY to bring forward the day when safety testing takes place using only human- based methods, without animals.

Past nominations have been welcomed from across Japan, South Korea, China, Taiwan, Singapore and Malaysia. In 2016, a record number of nominations 55 projects/scientists from 21 countries, including Japan, South Korea, China and Singapore [5]. The prize welcomes many future nominations from across the Asia region and worldwide.

Many initiatives are directed at the '3Rs': reduction, refinement, and replacement of the use of animals. The Lush Prize seeks only to support projects working on the genuine replacement of animal tests and is the largest reward in its field.

Nominations open for the Lush Prize open in March each year. Any individual(s) or organisation who wish to apply must submit a full nomination form by the June deadline. Judging is carried out by an independent panel of experts from around the world – scientists, lobbyists and campaigners. Winners participate in a conference and attend a prestigious awards ceremony. Full details of the Young Researcher Award [6] and other award categories are available on the Lush Prize website [1].

References

1. The lush prize (2017). http://lushprize.org/. Accessed 15 Dec 2017
2. OECD (Organisation for Economic Co-operation and Development) (2017). http://www.oecd.org/chemicalsafety/testing/oecdguidelinesforthetestingofchemicals.htm. Accessed 15 Dec 2017
3. The adverse outcome pathway for skin sensitisation initiated by covalent binding to proteins (2017). http://www.oecd.org/env/the-adverse-outcome-pathway-for-skin-sensitisation-initiated-by-covalent-binding-to-proteins-9789264221444-en.htm. Accessed 17 Dec 2017

4. Young researcher Asia (2016). http://lushprize.org/2016-prize/2016-young-researcher-asia. Accessed 17 Dec 2017
5. The lush prize; past years. http://www.lushprize.org/past-years/. Accessed 17 Dec 2017
6. Young researcher prize. http://www.lushprize.org/awards/young-researcher-prize/. Accessed 17 Dec 2017

Author Index

H. Kojima et al. (Eds.): *Alternatives to Animal Testing*, pp. 129–130, 2019.
https://doi.org/10.1007/978-981-13-2447-5

www.ingramcontent.com/pod-product-compliance
Lightning Source LLC
LaVergne TN
LVHW082237200926
848484LV00008B/2369